Promoting Executive Function in the Classroom

WHAT WORKS FOR SPECIAL-NEEDS LEARNERS
Karen R. Harris and Steve Graham
Editors

Strategy Instruction for Students with Learning Disabilities
Robert Reid and Torri Ortiz Lienemann

Teaching Mathematics to Middle School Students with Learning Difficulties
Marjorie Montague and Asha K. Jitendra, Editors

Teaching Word Recognition:
Effective Strategies for Students with Learning Difficulties
Rollanda E. O'Connor

Teaching Reading Comprehension to Students with Learning Difficulties
Janette K. Klingner, Sharon Vaughn, and Alison Boardman

Promoting Self-Determination in Students with Developmental Disabilities
*Michael L. Wehmeyer with Martin Agran, Carolyn Hughes,
James E. Martin, Dennis E. Mithaug, and Susan B. Palmer*

Instructional Practices for Students with Behavioral Disorders:
Strategies for Reading, Writing, and Math
J. Ron Nelson, Gregory J. Benner, and Paul Mooney

Working with Families of Young Children with Special Needs
R. A. McWilliam, Editor

Promoting Executive Function in the Classroom
Lynn Meltzer

Promoting Executive Function in the Classroom

Lynn Meltzer

Series Editor's Note by Karen R. Harris and Steve Graham

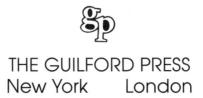

THE GUILFORD PRESS
New York   London

© 2010 The Guilford Press
A Division of Guilford Publications, Inc.
72 Spring Street, New York, NY 10012
www.guilford.com

Printed in the United States of America

This book is printed on acid-free paper.

Last digit is print number: 9   8   7   6   5   4   3   2   1

Library of Congress Cataloging-in-Publication Data

Meltzer, Lynn.
   Promoting executive function in the classroom / by Lynn Meltzer.
      p. cm.
   Includes bibliographical references and index.
   ISBN 978-1-60623-616-1 (pbk.: alk. paper)
   1.   Curriculum planning.   2.   Classroom management.   3.   Classroom environ-
ment.   I.   Title.
   LB3013.M397 2010
   371.3—dc22
                                                        2010002443

To Pete, for always being there to help navigate
the route to the top of the mountain
—L. M.

About the Author

Lynn Meltzer, PhD, is Co-Founder and Co-Director of the Institute for Learning and Development (ILD) and ResearchILD in Lexington, Massachusetts. She holds appointments as an Associate in Education at the Harvard Graduate School of Education and as an Adjunct Associate Professor in the Department of Child Development at Tufts University. She is a fellow and past President of the International Academy for Research in Learning Disabilities. Dr. Meltzer's over 30 years of experience in assessment and clinical consultation with children, adolescents, and adults emphasizes the critical importance of the theory-to-practice cycle of knowledge. Her research, publications, and presentations have focused on understanding the complexity of learning and attention problems, using a multidimensional model to bridge the gap between theory, research, and practice. Her extensive publications and professional presentations include articles, chapters, and books relating to the assessment and treatment of learning difficulties, with an emphasis on the importance of metacognition, strategy use, cognitive flexibility, self-concept, and resilience. Dr. Meltzer is the founder and chair of the Annual Learning Differences Conference, now in its 25th year at the Harvard Graduate School of Education. She is on the editorial boards of several prestigious education journals. Her recent work with her ResearchILD colleagues includes books for professionals (*Strategies for Success*, 2006) and parents (*Parent Guide to Hassle-Free Homework*, 2007) and two award-winning interactive software products (BrainCogs and Essay Express), all with an emphasis on teaching critical executive function and learning strategies. Her most recent edited book (*Executive Function in Education: From Theory to Practice*, 2007) addresses our current understanding of executive function processes.

Contributing Authors

Jennifer Sage Bagnato, MEd, works as an educational diagnostician at the Stern Center for Language and Learning in Williston, Vermont, where she provides comprehensive evaluations and direct instruction to middle and high school students. Prior to joining the Stern Center, she was an educational specialist at the Institute for Learning and Development (ILD) and ResearchILD in Lexington, Massachusetts, and an elementary and middle school teacher for over 15 years.

Surina Basho, MA, is an educational specialist at ILD and ResearchILD. She is also a doctoral student in the Department of Child Development at Tufts University. She has extensive research experience in developmental cognitive neuroscience and applied educational research in executive function. Ms. Basho's clinical experience includes conducting comprehensive psychoeducational assessments and providing individualized educational therapy for middle and high school students with learning differences and attentional issues.

Jason Bendezu, BS, is a graduate student at Tufts University and an intern at ResearchILD in Lexington, Massachusetts, where he is involved in the ongoing SMARTS Leadership and Mentoring Program. His work focuses on studying and evaluating the impact of SMARTS Boston, an ongoing program in the inner-city schools for students who are at risk academically and socially. Mr Bendezu develops qualitative procedures for measuring the extent to which SMARTS is meeting its goals of building motivation, resilience, and proactivity in students. Additionally, he helps ensure the program's efficacy through ongoing on-site data collection and analysis.

Melissa J. Feller, MS, CCC-SLP, is a speech–language pathologist and reading specialist at ILD and ResearchILD in Lexington, Massachusetts, where she conducts comprehensive evaluations of children and adolescents with communication, learning, and attention differences. She also provides individualized speech–language and educational therapy to children and adolescents, addressing needs in speech, language, reading/writing, executive function processes, and math. Prior to joining ResearchILD, Ms. Feller provided speech–language therapy and specialized reading instruction to middle school students with a variety of speech, language, and learning difficulties.

Lena Hannus-Suksi, MA, is a special educator living and working in Turku, Finland. From 2008 to 2009, she worked as a volunteer at ResearchILD in Lexington, Massachusetts. Ms. Hannus-Suksi is now a special educator in a Swedish-speaking middle school in Turku, and is involved in the assessment and remediation of mostly bilingual students with various learning differences. She is a board member of the Finnish affiliate of the International Reading Association.

Donna M. Kincaid, MEd, is an educational specialist and training coordinator at ILD and ResearchILD in Lexington, Massachusetts. She conducts comprehensive psychoeducational assessments and provides individual educational therapy for middle and high school students with learning and attentional issues. Her 30 years of experience in the field of special education include teaching, supervising, testing, consulting, professional development, and administrative responsibilities. In the public school sector, Ms. Kincaid has worked with all levels of professional staff, from teachers to superintendents.

Kalyani Krishnan, MA, is Assistant Director of Assessment and a language and learning specialist at ILD and ResearchILD in Lexington, Massachusetts. Over the past 15 years, she has worked with numerous students in her capacity as a clinician and teacher. She has consulted with families and schools, has taught graduate-level classes, and has been a presenter on numerous occasions at the Annual Learning Differences Conference at the Harvard Graduate School of Education. Ms. Krishnan has contributed to a number of recent books with her ResearchILD colleagues, including *Executive Function in Education: From Theory to Practice* (2007) and *Parent Guide to Hassle-Free Homework* (2007).

Melissa Orkin, MA, is a doctoral student in the Department of Child Development at Tufts University and a research assistant at the Tufts Center for Reading and Language Research. Ms. Orkin has worked in schools, clinical settings, and the nonprofit sector as a remedial reading teacher, a curriculum designer, an educational therapist, and a diagnostician.

Laura Sales Pollica, MA, is an educational specialist at ILD and ResearchILD in Lexington, Massachusetts, where she is involved in assessment, remediation, and research addressing the needs of students with a wide range of learning differences. Her work with students focuses on teaching strategies for executive function, math, written expression, and reading. Ms. Sales Pollica codeveloped the *Master Your Mind* summer course for middle and high school students, which teaches students strategies to foster their executive function processes in academic and nonacademic areas. In addition, she has contributed to a number of recent books, including *Executive Function in Education: From Theory to Practice* (2007) and *Parent Guide to Hassle-Free Homework* (2007).

Wendy Stacey, MS, is a reading and learning disability specialist at ILD and ResearchILD in Lexington, Massachusetts, and a certified special educator. She assesses and teaches students with language-based learning disabilities and provides consultation services to surrounding public and private schools. As a researcher with the *Drive to Thrive* project, she helped design and teach test-taking strategies to students. Ms. Stacey coauthored a language arts curriculum to meet both the general Massachusetts standards and the needs of students with language-based learning disabilities. She has also taught oral expression and language arts to elementary and middle school students at the Landmark School in Prides Crossing, Massachusetts, and literature and composition to adolescents at the Carroll School in Lincoln, Massachusetts, both private schools for students with specific language-based learning disabilities.

Judith A. Stein, PhD, is Coordinator of Clinical Services at ILD and ResearchILD in Lexington, Massachusetts, where she provides individual and group therapy for children and adults, comprehensive neuropsychological assessments, social skills training for children, school consultations, and parent education. Her special interests are working with children with learning and attentional problems, treating anxiety and mood disorders, and providing consultations in the area of nonverbal learning disorders. Most recently, Dr. Stein has been involved in training and supervising mentors in ResearchILD's innovative SMARTS Leadership and Mentoring Program. She is also a contributing author to ResearchILD's most recent publications, *Parent Guide to Hassle-Free Homework* (2007) and *Executive Function in Education: From Theory to Practice* (2007).

Nancy Trautman, MAT, is an educational specialist at ILD and ResearchILD in Lexington, Massachusetts, and a certified Orton–Gillingham specialist. She provides educational therapy and assessments to elementary, middle, and high school students with learning and attention problems and specializes in improving reading fluency, reading comprehension, writing, and math. Ms. Trautman also provides students with strategy instruction and individualized coaching in study skills, with an emphasis on teaching executive function processes.

Series Editors' Note

Executive function processes such as planning, organizing, prioritizing, and self-checking are critical to children's school performance. Yet, until now, there has not been a book that provides step-by-step instructions and practical tools for developing these strategies in the classroom. This book—filled with assessment tools, teaching techniques, and reproducibles—provides concrete ways to integrate executive function in the curriculum, including specific examples in the context of teaching reading, writing, and math. Lynn Meltzer and her team at ResearchILD are in the forefront of this field and bring a wealth of current knowledge and experience to show how teachers can actively evaluate which students need help, while also giving students the skills and strategies they need to help themselves.

This book is part of the series What Works for Special-Needs Learners. While researchers in special education, educational psychology, curriculum and instruction, and other fields have made great progress in understanding what works for struggling learners, the practical application of this research base remains quite limited. Books in the series present assessment, instructional, and classroom management methods that have strong empirical evidence. Written in a user-friendly format, each volume provides specific how-to instructions and examples of the use of proven procedures in schools.

KAREN R. HARRIS
STEVE GRAHAM

Preface

Ben has the ability but not the desire. He is always late for class, and he can never find his books or papers in his backpack. When I assign a new long-term assignment, he usually has wonderful ideas. However, his papers are often incomplete, and he never hands in the final project on time. His grades are always lower than they should be because his work is always late. His grades can jump from 50% to 90% in one week. I wish he would apply himself.

—SEVENTH-GRADE TEACHER

In our technologically oriented 21st-century society, academic success is increasingly dependent on students' ability to plan their time, organize, prioritize, distinguish main ideas from details, shift approaches flexibly, monitor their own progress, and reflect on their work. From the elementary grades onward, these executive function processes affect many academic areas and are critically important for reading comprehension, written language, math problem solving, long-term projects, studying, and taking tests. These processes are not taught systematically in schools and are not a focus of the curriculum, which typically emphasizes competency and efficiency in the traditional "three R's"—reading, writing, and arithmetic. In fact, classroom instruction tends to emphasize the content, or *what*, of learning rather than the process, or *how*, of learning even though teachers require students to complete long-term projects, lengthy writing assignments, and open-book tests that rely heavily on executive function processes. Because many students are inefficient with their work, and their academic performance does not seem to match their potential, they are viewed by their teachers as "lazy," "unmotivated," "disorganized," "unprepared," or "not very smart." As a result, all students, and especially those with learning and/or attention difficulties, will benefit from explicit instruction that systematically embeds selected executive function processes in the different content areas.

The purpose of this book is to provide teachers with practical suggestions for scaffolding the teaching of selected executive function processes into the classroom curriculum. My colleagues and I discuss the rationale, as well as specific suggestions, for implementing classroom-based strategy instruction that systematically addresses many of the key executive function processes. Particular emphasis is placed on the importance of differentiating strategy instruction to address the needs of students with learning and/or attention difficulties. Chapters include practical strategies for targeting selected executive function processes that are the focus of this book, namely, planning, organizing, accessing working memory, shifting approaches flexibly, and self-checking. We also address the influence of emotional self-regulation on students' attention, engagement, and working memory, and their willingness to make the effort to use executive function strategies in the classroom. There is also a discussion of the cyclical relationship that connects these executive function processes with motivation, effort, self-awareness, and persistence—all attributes that build resilience and academic success. It should be noted that it is beyond the scope of this book to provide a detailed discussion of the impact of inhibitory control, selective attention, and activation, all important executive function processes that are emphasized in neuroscientific research (Anderson, Rani Jacobs, & Anderson, 2008; Bernstein & Waber, 2007; Diamond, 2006).

All the chapters in this book emphasize practical suggestions for creating "strategic classrooms" that address the needs of a wide range of learners, particularly struggling students with learning and/or attention problems. Some of these strategies have been evaluated in our school-based *Gateways to Success* and *Drive to Thrive* studies with thousands of students in six different school systems (Meltzer, Katzir, Miller, Reddy, & Roditi, 2004a; Meltzer, Reddy, Sales Pollica, & Roditi, 2004b; Meltzer et al., 2004c); others stem from extensive clinical research (Meltzer, Roditi, Steinberg, Biddle, Taber, Caron, & Kniffin, 2006; Meltzer, Sales Pollica, & Barzillai, 2007b); and yet others represent best practice. Nevertheless, caution should be exercised in interpreting and implementing these suggestions and strategies, which have not yet been comprehensively evaluated in longitudinal studies. Rather, teachers should use them as guides for developing their own approaches to teaching strategies in the context of their classroom curricula.

In Part I, we focus on the challenges faced by 21st-century teachers as they grapple with the complexities involved in understanding the impact of executive function processes on students' academic performance. In Part II, we discuss ways of scaffolding teaching strategies into the daily curriculum, given the time pressure teachers face in covering the extensive amount of content imposed by standards-based testing. The same organizational framework is used in Chapters 3–8 of Part II, so that there is consistency, flow, and coherence within and across chapters. Specifically, each of these chapters includes sections that focus on the *why, what,* and *how* of teaching strategies addressing five of the important executive function processes. These chapters also include specific examples for embedding these strategies into the academic domains of reading, written language, math, studying, and test taking.

In Chapter 1, I discuss a paradigm for understanding and teaching executive function processes to help close the gap that currently separates students' skills and strategies from the demands of school and the workplace. In Chapter 2, Surina

Basho and I provide an overview of the major principles that underlie the creation of "strategic classrooms" and a classroomwide culture that scaffolds the teaching of selected executive function processes into the daily curriculum. This chapter also focuses on how to create strategic classrooms, as well as what specific executive function processes can be embedded into content areas such as reading, writing, and math. Finally, there is a discussion of peer tutoring and peer mentoring in the classroom as ways of increasing motivation and engagement in all students.

In Part II, as noted above, we discuss ways of scaffolding teaching strategies into the daily curriculum. In Chapter 3, Kalyani Krishnan, Melissa J. Feller, and Melissa Orkin address the executive function processes of goal setting, planning, prioritizing, and managing time, as well as strategies for supporting and fostering the development of these processes within and across classrooms. They propose an approach for teaching these strategies that progresses developmentally from the elementary level (where the strategies are heavily modeled) to the middle school level (which promotes and teaches independence) to the secondary school level (where independence is supported). This same developmental sequence underlies the discussion in Chapter 4, where Kalyani Krishnan and Melissa J. Feller address strategies for helping students to organize their materials and their learning environment, as well as strategies for organizing expository and narrative information. In Chapter 5, Donna M. Kincaid and Nancy Trautman focus on approaches for teaching students how to retain and mentally manipulate information, with specific emphasis on working memory and automatic memory. They discuss strategies for improving students' ability to retain needed information and to retrieve facts, processes, and concepts so that they can learn efficiently. It should be noted that this chapter addresses working memory, in particular, and also emphasizes memory strategies that are broader, given the heavy learning–memory load imposed on students in our 21st-century information-driven classes. In Chapter 6, Jennifer Sage Bagnato and I discuss one of the least understood executive function processes: cognitive flexibility, or the ability to shift mindsets. We also provide strategies that teachers can implement in their classrooms to help their students shift mindsets and approaches flexibly in both classwork and homework. In Chapter 7, Jennifer Sage Bagnato and I discuss suggestions for helping students to self-monitor, self-check, and self-correct their work systematically. We emphasize that students' willingness to monitor themselves and check their own work is associated with their metacognitive awareness, as well as with their ability to shift flexibly from the final product of their efforts to the goals of the task. We also suggest techniques that students can use for shifting back and forth from the product to the process in order to recognize and correct their errors. In Chapter 8, Judith A. Stein discusses the critical importance of emotional self-regulation and impulse control for effective learning. She addresses the impact of emotional self-regulation on students' attention, retrieval, and problem solving in the classroom setting. She also emphasizes specific strategies that teachers and other professionals can use to help students develop more effective ways of managing their emotions.

In Part III, Lena Hannus-Suksi, Laura Sales Pollica, Wendy Stacey, Melissa J. Feller, and Jason Bendezu provide brief case vignettes that highlight particular students' difficulties with five key executive function processes and the impact on classroom performance. Summary tables focus on academic difficulties that students often display and ways of addressing these weaknesses through individual instruction and remediation and classroom accommodations. Finally, several practical, easy-to-use strategy worksheets are provided in the Appendix for use by teachers on a daily basis.

We hope that the suggestions provided in this book will stimulate teachers to develop their own solutions to the questions we have attempted to address:

- How can we create a school culture that fosters strategic mindsets in students from the first grade onward and that generalizes across grade levels?
- How can we create classrooms where executive function processes are taught systematically in the context of a curriculum that provides the sustained support that all students need?
- How can a differentiated instruction model incorporate the teaching of selected executive function processes such as goal setting, planning, organizing, prioritizing, and time management?
- How can teachers sustain and build students' motivation, so that students make the effort to use appropriate executive function strategies in their daily work?
- How can teachers create opportunities for academic success for students with learning and/or attention difficulties, so that the students feel self-confident and are willing to persist and make the effort to use executive function strategies?
- What systems and strategies are needed to help students whose anxiety compromises their ability to access executive function processes in order to manage the demands of the school day?

We also hope that this book helps teachers to create classrooms that promote thinking, reasoning, problem solving, and lifelong success, as reflected in Albert Einstein's comment: "Know where to find the information and how to use it—that's the secret of success."

LYNN MELTZER

Acknowledgments

I would like to thank a number of people whose support has been critical for the completion of this book. First, my appreciation to my long-time colleague and friend Bethany Roditi for her unwavering support, creative approach, and ongoing encouragement over the course of the planning, organization, and execution of this book. Thanks too to the wonderful staff and interns at the Research Institute for Learning and Development (ResearchILD) for their willingness to help with the many executive function processes involved in completing this book. I am particularly grateful to Laura Sales Pollica for her many excellent ideas and her help with developing, editing, and designing the charts and figures. A special thanks to those staff and interns who were willing to help with brainstorming, developing the case studies, editing our manuscript, and offering many wonderful suggestions—in particular, Andrew Porter, Kathy Button, Joan Steinberg, Lynn Gray, Mayumi Fei, Tia Bassano, Jason Bendezu, Andy Vosslamber, and Maia Noeder. Thanks too to Thelma Segal, for her dedication and expert help with editing, revising, and checking our manuscript. The help of our core ResearchILD staff, especially Mimi Ballard and Karen Caires, also made a major difference to the completion of this book. The support of the ResearchILD Board of Directors, especially Neil Motenko, Chair; Scott Barrie, Vice Chair; and Dave Caruso, Andrea Masterman, Elizabeth Brach, and Narain Bhatia, committee directors, made this project possible, for which I am so appreciative. Finally, thanks to Thomas A. Feller for his creative artistic illustrations.

I am especially grateful to Karen R. Harris, Currey Ingram Professor of Special Education and Literacy at Vanderbilt University and coeditor of the What Works for Special-Needs Learners series, for her excellent suggestions, flexibility, and willingness to devote the time to review and edit the manuscript so carefully. A special thanks to Rochelle Serwator, Senior Editor at The Guilford Press, for her unflagging enthusiasm as well as her ongoing commitment to excellence and to encouraging innovative ideas in education. Thanks, too, to Louise Farkas, Senior Production Editor, for her excellent editorial suggestions and her amazing attention to the numerous details involved in the production of this book. I am also grateful to Adele Diamond, Professor of Developmental Cognitive Neuroscience, University of British Columbia in Vancouver, Canada, for her many helpful suggestions and comments.

Finally, thanks to the many children, parents, and teachers whose persistence, determination, and resilience continue to inspire our work!

LYNN MELTZER

Contents

PART II. SCAFFOLDING EXECUTIVE FUNCTION PROCESSES INTO THE CURRICULUM CONTENT

8. Emotional Self-Regulation: A Critical Component   175
of Executive Function
JUDITH A. STEIN

PART III. CASE STUDIES: ADDRESSING EXECUTIVE FUNCTION WEAKNESSES ACROSS THE GRADES

LENA HANNUS-SUKSI, LAURA SALES POLLICA, WENDY STACEY,
MELISSA J. FELLER, and JASON BENDEZU

APPENDIX. REPRODUCIBLES FOR THE CLASSROOM

PART I

UNDERSTANDING EXECUTIVE FUNCTION

The Challenge for 21st-Century Teachers

CHAPTER 1

Understanding, Assessing, and Teaching Executive Function Processes

The Why, What, and How

LYNN MELTZER

> John is a puzzle to me. He seems so bright and creative, and he always contributes wonderful ideas to our class discussions. However, he often does not hand in homework, he does not seem to study for tests, and he is usually late with projects. I don't know if he is just lazy. I wish he was more motivated and invested in his work.
>
> —SIXTH-GRADE TEACHER

Academic success in the digital age is increasingly linked not only with students' technological expertise, but, even more important, with their mastery of such processes as goal setting, planning, prioritizing, organizing, shifting flexibly, holding/manipulating information in working memory, and self-monitoring. Collectively, these are termed *executive function* processes. Beginning in the early grades, students are now required to organize and integrate a rapidly changing body of information that is available through the Internet and to take greater responsibility for their own learning. Teachers give students lengthy reading and writing assignments, as well as long-term projects, that rely heavily on these executive function processes. Students are also expected to become proficient at note taking, studying, and test taking—all tasks that require the simultaneous organization and integration of multiple subskills. Academic success therefore depends on students' ability to plan and prioritize their time, organize materials and information, separate main ideas from details, shift approaches flexibly, monitor their own progress, and reflect on their work. As a result, it has become increasingly important for classroom teachers to teach strategies that address executive function processes systematically, in order to help students understand *how* they think and *how* they learn.

This chapter provides a paradigm for understanding and teaching students strategies that address executive function processes. The chapter also begins to describe how to address the needs of the increasing numbers of students who exhibit major weaknesses in such processes. These students benefit from explicit and systematic strategy instruction, as well as from accommodations for classwork and homework. There is a focus on five major themes:

1. *What* is executive function, and how do selected executive function processes affect academic performance?
2. *Why* are executive function processes so important?
3. *How* can teachers begin to understand and informally assess students' executive function processes?
4. *How* can teachers address the needs of students with executive function weaknesses?
5. *How* can core strategies be taught across tasks, content areas, and grades?

WHAT IS EXECUTIVE FUNCTION, AND HOW DO EXECUTIVE FUNCTION PROCESSES AFFECT ACADEMIC PERFORMANCE?

> I sit down and my mind feels like there's a hurricane building.
> I grab an idea . . . if I can think of three good sentences, I go
> with it. If not, I find another idea.
> —JOHN, EIGHTH GRADER

Until recently, studies of executive function processes have primarily been the domain of neurologists and neuropsychologists, who have emphasized the importance of the prefrontal cortex in controlling these processes and the behaviors that are affected by them (Anderson, Rani, Jacobs, & Anderson, 2008; Denckla, 1996; Diamond, 2006; Holmes Bernstein & Waber, 2007). Over the past several years, educators have begun to recognize the importance of executive function processes for educational performance. This shift is due in part to clinicians' efforts to explain why so many extremely bright students fail to perform at the level of their potential, and why certain students present as "poor students" despite their strong performance on short, highly structured, standardized measures (Denckla, 2005, 2007; Meltzer, 2007). In fact, weak executive function processes are often associated with such students' academic difficulties, and especially with the problems they experience in deploying and coordinating the many skills needed for such tasks as open-ended projects, term papers, and tests.

Executive function processes can be explained by using the analogy of a mountaintop view (Meltzer, 2007, 2008a, 2008b) (see Figures 1.1a and 1.1b). A person standing at the top of a mountain has a bird's eye-view of the entire panorama spread out below—in other words, an overview of the "big picture." Standing at the bottom of the mountain, the viewer only sees thousands of leaves on individual

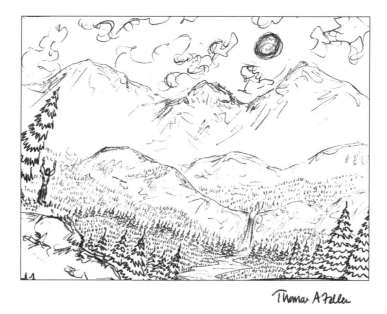

FIGURE 1.1a. The panoramic view from the mountaintop allows students to focus on the major themes or the "big picture."

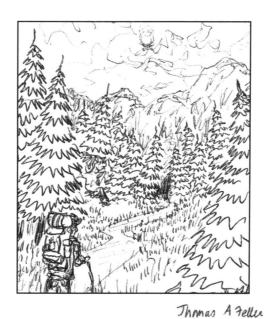

FIGURE 1.1b. From the bottom of the mountain, there is only a view of individual trees.

trees. Executive function processes allow the viewer to shift back and forth flexibly between the big picture seen from the mountaintop and the numerous details seen from the bottom of the mountain.

Just as they do for the viewer on the mountaintop, executive function processes help students to understand the "big picture" or major themes as well as the relevant details and to shift back and forth between the two. In this book, we discuss practical suggestions that teachers can implement to address five key executive function processes: goal setting, planning, and prioritizing; organizing; retaining and manipulating information in working memory; shifting flexibly; and self-monitoring/self-checking (Meltzer, 2007, 2008a, 2008b; Meltzer & Krishnan, 2007). These executive function processes are critically important for all aspects of academic performance.[1] Table 1.1 gives both formal and "student-friendly" definitions for several of these processes, as well as examples.

Because so many academic tasks require the coordination and integration of multiple subskills, as well as the ability to shift back and forth from the themes to the details, executive function weaknesses can have a significant impact on the accuracy and efficiency of students' performance. Writing, summarizing, note taking, and reading complex text for meaning may be particularly challenging for students with such weaknesses, whose struggle to produce can be explained by using the analogy of a clogged funnel. This analogy for understanding the impact of weak executive function processes on academic performance is illustrated in

TABLE 1.1. Examples of Several Key Executive Function Processes

Process	Definition	Example
Prioritizing	Ordering based on relative importance *Figuring out what's most important*	Ordering information for written work, projects, and tests Separating main ideas from details on reading and writing tasks
Organizing	Arranging information, systematizing *Moving and sorting information*	Using charts and graphic organizers for writing Using maps and webs for reading and writing
Using working memory	Manipulating information mentally *Juggling information in the brain*	Taking notes; completing multistep projects; completing math calculations mentally; thinking about themes while reading.
Shifting	Switching easily between approaches *Looking again, in a brand-new way*	Predicting different endings for novels Understanding different word meanings in text Applying different problem-solving approaches to word problems
Self-monitoring/ Self-checking	Reviewing work for common errors *Recognizing and fixing the most common kinds of mistakes*	Using personalized checklists Shifting to a checking mindset and back

Note. Italics indicate "student-friendly" definitions.

---

[1]Strategies for addressing the other executive function processes such as inhibition, selective attention, and activation, are beyond the scope of this book.

Figure 1.2 (Meltzer, 2007, 2008a, 2008b; Meltzer & Krishnan, 2007). As is evident from this figure, students with executive function difficulties often experience an overload of information, so that input exceeds output. They struggle to plan, organize, and prioritize, with the result that information becomes clogged in the top of the funnel. Because these students cannot process this information rapidly enough and cannot shift approaches flexibly, they cannot easily unclog the funnel to produce finished work.

For students with executive function weaknesses, therefore, their conceptual reasoning abilities may be stronger than their output and productivity. Consequently, these students are inefficient with their work and have difficulty showing what they know in the classroom; their study skills and test performance are compromised; and their academic grades may not reflect their actual intellectual ability. As these students enter middle and high school, their difficulties become more evident, due to the mismatch between their skills and the curriculum demands. They have particular problems with academic tasks that involve the coordination and integration of different subskills, such as getting started on writing assignments; summarizing information; taking notes; studying; planning, executing, and completing projects in a timely manner; sustaining attention during long, detailed assignments and remembering to submit their work on time (see Table 1.2 for more specific examples). Furthermore, their problems with attention, working memory, and inhibition create additional challenges, and their productivity with classwork and homework is affected.

Students therefore need to understand their own learning styles. This will help them to discover which strategies work well for them, as well as *why, where, when,* and *how* to apply each specific strategy. This understanding is referred to as

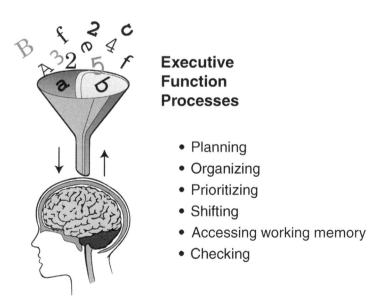

Executive Function Processes

- Planning
- Organizing
- Prioritizing
- Shifting
- Accessing working memory
- Checking

FIGURE 1.2. Executive function: The funnel model. From Meltzer and Krishnan (2007). Copyright 2007 by The Guilford Press. Reprinted by permission.

TABLE 1.2. Common Difficulties Experienced by Students with Executive Function Weaknesses

Planning

- Planning and allocating time to the many steps involved in different assignments (e.g., writing papers, taking notes for history or science, or completing long-term projects).

Prioritizing

- Prioritizing by allocating more time and effort to major projects and tests.
- Figuring out which details are critical and which details can be ignored when reading, taking notes, or writing essays.
- Estimating how much time to spend on reading and research versus output (e.g., writing a paper, editing, and layout).

Organizing

- Organizing ideas, such as summarizing key ideas on strategy cards rather than rereading the text over and over.
- Organizing materials such as class notes, textbooks, and study guides.
- Organizing workspace (e.g., reducing distractions and clutter).

Shifting

- Shifting flexibly from the major themes to the relevant details to meet the demands of the reading, writing, or studying task.
- Using outlines such as graphic organizers or linear outlines to get "unstuck" when writing papers or projects.
- Shifting between operations and between words and numbers for math computation or word problems.

Accessing Working Memory

- Studying strategically so that complex information is retained over time to prevent the "Friday spelling test effect" (Meltzer et.al., 2006). Here, students remember facts and spelling for quizzes and tests, but do not connect concepts and cannot juggle the information mentally so they can access this information on a long-term basis.
- Remembering to hand in completed assignments on time (e.g., students with executive function difficulties often leave school with their homework still in their bags).
- Remembering to bring necessary books and materials from school to home and back again.
- Keeping in mind the importance of remembering to check and correct "careless errors" when writing papers, taking tests, or doing homework.
- Performing consistently across situations, content areas, and tasks.

metacognition, or the ability to think about one's own thinking and learning. Metacognition underlies students' use of executive function processes and is discussed further in the next two sections of this chapter.

WHY ARE EXECUTIVE FUNCTION PROCESSES SO IMPORTANT?

> My success is due to the strategies I learned, as well as
> my self-understanding and the confidence I developed
> after I used the strategies and got higher grades.
> —Sean, 11th grader

Academic success for all students, and particularly for students with learning difficulties, is inextricably linked with their motivation, effort, persistence, academic self-concept, and self-efficacy (Brunstein, Schultheiss, & Grassman, 1998; Helliwell,

2003; Kasser & Ryan, 1996; Meltzer, Reddy, Sales Pollica, & Roditi, 2004b; Pajares & Schunk, 2001; Sheldon & Elliot, 1999). These cognitive and motivational processes are connected cyclically with students' use of executive function strategies, as well as with their academic performance (Meltzer et al., 2004b; Meltzer & Krishnan, 2007). As is evident from Figure 1.3, strategies that address executive function processes provide an entry point for improving academic performance. When students learn and apply these strategies effectively, they become more efficient and thus begin to succeed academically. Academic success in turn boosts self-confidence and academic self-concept, which results in more focused effort so that students' hard work is targeted strategically toward specific goals. In this way, a cycle of success is promoted (Meltzer, Katzir, Miller, Reddy, & Roditi, 2004a; Meltzer et al., 2004b; Meltzer et al., 2004c).

The learning environment and the instructional methods/materials all play an important role in mediating this cyclical relationship. For all students, but particularly for students with learning and/or attention difficulties, effective strategies and focused effort will help them to bridge gaps between their skills and the academic demands they face (Graham & Harris, 2003; Swanson, Harris, & Graham, 2003; Swanson & Hoskyn, 2001). In other words, their academic performance is often dependent on their knowledge of and willingness to use strategies. Maintaining the effort and hard work needed to master and implement strategies is often a major struggle for students with learning and attention difficulties (Meltzer & Krishnan, 2007). In fact, they may need to work much longer hours than their peers, and their grades may not reflect their effort. When these students use strategies for organizing, prioritizing, and checking, they are often able to bypass their deficits and to shift flexibly among different approaches and mindsets. When they select meaningful and realistic goals, make the effort needed to attain these goals, and self-regulate their cognitive and emotional processes, they

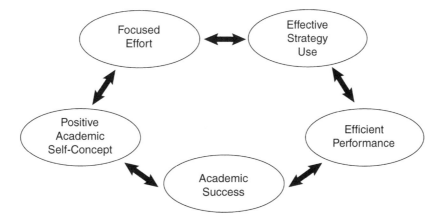

FIGURE 1.3. Academic success cycle. From Meltzer, Reddy, Sales Pollica, and Roditi (2004b). Copyright 2004 by the International Academy for Research in Learning Disabilities. Reprinted by permission.

usually succeed (Raskind, Goldberg, Higgins, & Herman, 1999) (See Chapters, 3, 4, and 8).

To build their motivation, persistence, and work ethic, students need to understand their profiles of strengths and weaknesses. Doing so enables them to determine which strategies work well for them, as well as *why, where, when*, and *how* to apply specific strategies. As noted above, this understanding is known as *metacognition*, or the ability to think about own's own thinking and learning. More specifically, metacognition, as defined originally by Flavell (1979) and Brown, Bransford, Ferrara, and Campione (1983), refers to each student's understanding and beliefs about how he or she learns, as well as the strategies that can or should be used to accomplish specific tasks. Students' metacognitive awareness therefore includes their knowledge and understanding of their own learning profiles, as well as their understanding of those executive function strategies that match their strengths and weaknesses and help them to master different tasks. For example, students like Chace (see Figure 1.4) are aware of their struggles with organization, and they are often frustrated that their academic performance does not match their strong intellectual potential.

Students like Chace are more likely to make the effort needed to use strategies that help them to stay organized and focused when they develop metacognitive awareness and are highly motivated to succeed and meet their goals. In other words, students' understanding of their strengths and weaknesses, as well as their motivation and beliefs, directly affect their selection of specific strategies and their willingness to persist with specific tasks. Beliefs about ability often span a number of areas, as discussed by Reid and Lienemann (2006):

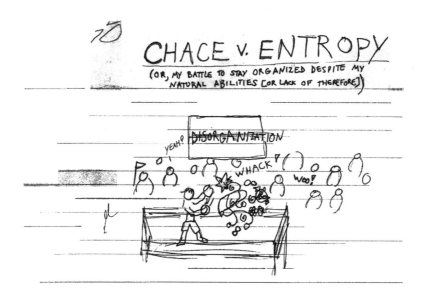

FIGURE 1.4. Chace, an exceptionally bright eighth grader, depicts his daily struggle to stay organized and focused as an ongoing battle because of his executive function difficulties.

- *General ability*: "How good am I as a learner? How smart am I?"
- *Competency on specific tasks*: "How good am I at this specific task (e.g., writing a report about the civil rights movement)?"
- *Control over outcomes*: "Can I control how well I do? If I work hard on this task, will I do well?"
- *Causes of failure*: "Why did I succeed or fail? Did I succeed because I worked hard and used appropriate strategies on this task?"
- *Understanding the benefits of specific strategies*: "Did I do well because I used specific organizational and self-checking strategies?"

When students can answer such questions, they reach a better understanding of the match between their own learning profiles and specific strategies, and thus become more likely to persist in acquiring and using these strategies. They are also more likely to make the extraordinary effort needed to apply the strategies to the many open-ended academic tasks that they face in school on a daily basis. Sustaining this major effort is often dependent on students' passions, as well as their interest in particular subjects. Specifically, interest-based motivation in learning frequently influences the kinds of strategies students use, as well as their learning outcomes (Hidi, Renninger, & Krapp, 2004; Yun Dai & Sternberg, 2004). Students' interest in school often begins to decrease as early as first grade (Renninger et al., 2004). There is an even steeper decline in middle and high school, when the curriculum content constrains students' ability to engage their interests and explore new challenges (Gardner, 1983; Hidi et al., 2004). As a result, many bright and talented students with learning and attention difficulties may "give up" and become unproductive in the later grades. At this time, their limited interest in the curriculum content is no longer strong enough to harness their motivation to expend the often superhuman effort needed to master the academic demands. For these students, executive function strategies can provide a lifeline to academic success.

HOW CAN TEACHERS BEGIN TO UNDERSTAND STUDENTS' EXECUTIVE FUNCTION STRENGTHS AND WEAKNESSES?

> I am a hard worker and I am not the best, nor am I a miracle worker.
> —JAMIE, EIGHTH GRADER

> My teacher probably thinks I am one taco short of a combo plate, if you know what I mean.
> —JAMIE, EIGHTH GRADER

> Jamie is a very bright student who is a puzzle to me. He does well on quizzes and short tests, but he often does not hand in his homework. His performance is inconsistent, and his grades are up and down.
> —JAMIE, EIGHTH-GRADE TEACHER

Teachers are often puzzled by the inconsistent performance of students like Jamie, who attain high grades on specific, short-term tasks (e.g., quizzes), but under-achieve on more demanding tasks (e.g., written reports, essays, math problem solving, long-term projects, or tests that span a broad content area). When teachers understand the role of executive function processes, they can more easily recognize the extent to which students like Jamie may struggle to perform adequately on open-ended tasks or tasks that require the coordination and integration of multiple skills and strategies. This context can help teachers to reframe their understanding of their students with executive function difficulties, so that they focus on these students' strengths and academic potential, rather than viewing them as "unmotivated," "lazy," or "not trying hard enough." Classroom-based assessment measures can help teachers to understand their students' strengths and weaknesses, and to determine whether students' difficulties fall within the "normal range" or are problematic and need referrals for assessment. (As shown in Figure 1.5, it is often helpful to compare students' own descriptions of their learning styles, and their perceptions of how their parents or teachers might describe their learning styles, with the parents' or teachers' actual descriptions.) A few specific assessment approaches that teachers can use are discussed below.

HOW CAN TEACHERS INFORMALLY ASSESS EXECUTIVE FUNCTION?

Teachers' insights about students' specific difficulties and their input into the assessment process are critically important. In fact, teachers are often informal diagnosticians who rely on their observations as well as on a variety of classroom-based assessment methods—a process we (Meltzer, 1993; Roditi, 1993) have referred to as *assessment for teaching* (AFT; see Figure 1.6). In this regard, informal assessment methods help teachers to understand students' use of executive function processes and to pinpoint *why* and *how* particular students may be struggling. Performance-

---

Student's Self-Perceptions

• How would you describe yourself as a student?
  "A very organized student and a good listener."

• How do you think your teachers would describe you as a student?
  "Pretty neat and a pretty good listener."

Teacher's Perceptions

• What words would come to mind to describe this student (e.g., motivated, hard-working, invested)?
  "Distracted, curious, eager to please, fidgety, impulsive."

FIGURE 1.5. Perceptions of Sally, a sixth grader who views herself as a good student, compared with her teacher's perceptions of her.

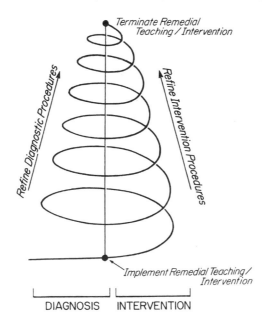

FIGURE 1.6. The Assessment for Teaching (AFT) model.

based assessment and portfolio assessment (Fuchs & Fuchs, 1991) are examples of these types of classroom measures.

By implementing an AFT cycle, teachers access baseline information about their students' learning profiles that helps them to understand each student's level of metacognitive awareness, effort, and strategy use. Teachers can then introduce specific instructional approaches, assess students' progress, and modify instruction. The continuous cycle linking assessment and teaching allows teachers to adjust their instructional methods to the changing needs of their students. In fact, many of these principles are incorporated into the response to intervention (RTI) approach that has recently been introduced into schools (Fuchs & Fuchs, 1991; Kame'enui, 2007).

Currently, there is a dearth of measures teachers can use to understand their students' executive function processes, and teachers must often rely on their personal insights as well as information they acquire from their conferences with parents. The Behavior Rating Inventory of Executive Function (BRIEF; Gioia, Isquith, Guy, & Kenworthy, 2000; Gioia, Isquith, Kenworthy, & Barton, 2002) is a highly reliable and widely used questionnaire system that consists of multiple rating forms, a parent questionnaire, and a teacher questionnaire, as well as a self-rating form for students from 12 years into adulthood. The BRIEF includes 86 items that assess behaviors associated with the core executive function processes, such as "Forgets to hand in homework, even when completed," "Gets caught up in details and misses the big picture," "Becomes overwhelmed by large assignments," and "Underestimates the time needed to finish tasks."

Another criterion-referenced assessment system that compares students', teachers', and parents' perceptions of the students' metacognitive awareness and strategy use is the Metacognitive Awareness System (MetaCOG; Meltzer et al., 2004b; Meltzer & Krishnan, 2007; Miller, Meltzer, Katzir-Cohen, & Houser, 2001). The MetaCOG, for use with 9- to 18-year-olds, comprises five rating scales that allow teachers to compare their own judgments with their students' self-ratings of their effort, strategy use, and academic performance (see Table 1.3). These strategy ratings focus on academic areas that depend on executive function processes, including written language, homework, studying, and taking tests (Meltzer, Katzir-Cohen, Miller, & Roditi, 2001; Miller et al., 2001).

As is evident from Table 1.3 and the descriptions that follow, the three student surveys assess students' self-ratings of their motivation and effort, as well as their strategy use in key academic areas. The two teacher surveys include similar questions, so that a direct comparison can be drawn between students' and teachers' ratings. Teachers can use these questionnaires at the beginning of the school year to gain an understanding of how much effort students think they put into their work, how often they use strategies, and how well they think they perform academically (Meltzer & Krishnan, 2007). Teachers can also discuss students' self-ratings on these surveys at parent conferences, so that parents and teachers can gain shared insights into students' views of the importance of hard work and academic success.

MetaCOG Student Surveys

Motivation and Effort Survey

The Motivation and Effort Survey (ME) consists of 38 items asking for students' self-ratings of their effort and performance on different academic tasks that depend on executive function processes (alpha = .91) (Meltzer et al., 2004c; Meltzer, Sayer, Sales, Theokas, & Roditi, 2002). Sample items are shown in Figure 1.7. Students rate themselves on a 1–5 scale (from "never" to "always") in terms of how hard they work and how well they do in selected academic areas, such as reading, writing, math, homework, studying for tests, and long-term projects. They are also required to describe themselves as students.

TABLE 1.3. Components of the Metacognitive Awareness System (MetaCOG)

Student questionnaires
- ME—Motivation and Effort Survey
- STRATUS—Strategy Use Survey
- MAQ—Metacognitive Awareness Questionnaire

Teacher questionnaires
- TPSE—Teacher Perceptions of Student Effort
- TIQ—Teacher Information Questionnaire

5-point rating for all surveys

- I spend as much time as I need to get my work done.
- I finish my work even when it is boring.
- I do schoolwork before other things that are more fun.

FIGURE 1.7. Sample items from the Motivation and Effort Survey (ME): Students' ratings of their motivation and effort on a 1–5 scale.

Strategy Use Survey

The Strategy Use Survey (STRATUS) consists of 40 items that assess students' self-reported strategy use in reading, writing, spelling, math, studying, and test taking (alpha = .945). Items focus on students' perceptions of their use of planning, organizing, memorizing, shifting, and self-checking strategies for their schoolwork (see examples in Figure 1.8).

Metacognitive Awareness Questionnaire

The Metacognitive Awareness Questionnaire (MAQ) consists of 18 items that assess students' understanding of what strategies are and how they can apply strategies to their schoolwork (see examples in Figure 1.9). Students are also asked what they think a strategy is both before and after strategy instruction has occurred, to provide the teacher with insights about the effectiveness of strategy instruction. As is shown in Figure 1.10, students like these eighth graders have a fairly good understanding of strategies.

- When I have to remember new things in school, I make up acronyms to help me.
- Before I write, I plan out my ideas in some way that works for me (outline, list, map).
- When I do math, I ask if my answers make sense.

FIGURE 1.8. Sample items from the Strategy Use Survey (STRATUS): Students' ratings of their strategy use on a 1–5 scale.

- When you begin something new, do you try to connect it to something you already know?
- When you begin something new, do you try to think about how long it will take and make sure you have enough time?

FIGURE 1.9. Sample items from the Metacognitive Awareness Questionnaire (MAQ): Students' ratings of their understanding of strategies on a 1–5 scale.

What do you think a strategy is?

- A strategy is something that helps you remember something hard, like the Preamble to the Constitution or biology terms.
- A strategy is a way to help people order and organize things to prepare for a test. Also, it's a good shortcut because it helps, but it isn't cheating and it's fun.
- A strategy is something to help you write a long paper where you need to brainstorm to figure out what is most important.

FIGURE 1.10. Examples of eighth graders' definitions of a strategy.

MetaCOG Teacher Surveys

Teacher Perceptions of Student Effort

The Teacher Perceptions of Student Effort (TPSE) survey consists of 38 items that assess teachers' ratings of students' effort in different academic domains (alpha = .980) (Meltzer et al., 2004a, 2004b, 2004c). Teachers rate students' effort and performance in reading, writing, math, homework, tests, and long-term projects—all academic tasks that rely on executive function processes (see Figure 1.11 for sample items). Teachers also rate students' overall strategy use and academic performance in response to this question: "If you had to assign a grade for this student's overall academic performance, what would this be?"

Teacher Information Questionnaire

The Teacher Information Questionnaire (TIQ) assesses teachers' understanding of the terms *metacognitive, strategy,* and *effort,* as well as their understanding of effective ways for promoting students' strategy use and executive function processes in the classroom (see Figure 1.12 for sample items). Completion of this survey at the beginning of the school year helps teachers to reflect about their teaching philosophy and practices, and to develop an awareness of the importance of addressing executive function processes.

- S/he spends as much time as needed to get his/her work done.
- S/he does not give up even when the work is difficult.

FIGURE 1.11. Sample Items from the Teacher Perceptions of Student Effort (TPSE): Teachers' ratings of students' effort and strategy use on a 1–5 scale.

- Students use strategies effectively without being taught these strategies directly.
- Teaching the curriculum is more important than teaching strategies.
- It is possible to motivate every student to work hard.

FIGURE 1.12. Sample Items from the Teacher Information Questionnaire (TIQ): Teachers are asked their views about ways of teaching strategies effectively in the classroom (a 1–5 scale assesses the extent of their agreement or disagreement).

In summary, teachers can use survey systems such as the MetaCOG for a variety of purposes over the course of the year:

- To understand students' views of their own effort, use of strategies, and academic performance in the classroom.
- To develop a system for teaching strategies that help students plan, organize, prioritize, shift flexibly, memorize, and check their work.
- To help teachers understand their students' perceptions and judgments, and to compare their own views with their students' self-perceptions so that they can reach all their students and teach them to learn *how* to learn over the course of the school year.

Comparisons of Students' versus Teachers' Perceptions

As is evident from Tables 1.4a and 1.4b, teachers can directly compare their own perceptions with the views of their students, to help them plan their teaching and connect with each of their students. Students' perceptions of their own effort and strategy use are often very different from their parents' and teachers' perceptions, as has been shown in a number of studies (Meltzer et al., 2004a, 2004b, 2004c; Stone & May, 2002).

For example, Figure 1.13a (page 19) shows the self-ratings of John, a fifth grader. John rates himself as a strong student who works hard, with the goals of "getting a second master's degree" and "making the world a better place." When asked how his parents would describe him, his response reflects his parents' emphasis on the importance of working hard in school. When John's teacher is asked to judge his effort and performance, her comments reflect her perception that John has difficulty sustaining his attention and that his academic performance would be much stronger if he could focus.

A sixth-grade student named Lucy (whose self-ratings are shown in Figure 1.13b on page 19) views herself as very bright and hard-working, as does her teacher. However, her teacher also recognizes that Lucy's performance may be compromised by her organizational and attention difficulties.

TABLE 1.4a. Students' versus Teachers' Ratings of Their Motivation and Effort on Academic Tasks That Involve Executive Function Processes

ME—Students	TPSE—Teachers
• Doing well in school is important to me.	• Doing well in school is important to this student.
• I spend as much time as I need to get my work done.	• S/he is a hard worker.
• I keep working even when the work is difficult.	• S/he does not give up even when the work is difficult.
I work hard on:	*Please judge how hard this student works:*
• Homework	• Homework
• Long-term projects	• Long-term projects
• Studying for tests	• Studying for tests
• Other activities (sports, music, art, hobbies)	• Other activities (sports, music, art, hobbies)

Note. The ME and TPSE each comprise 36 items, which are rated on a 1–5 scale.

TABLE 1.4b. Students' versus Teachers' Ratings of Their Performance on Academic Tasks That Involve Executive Function Processes

ME—Students	TPSE—Teachers
Please judge how well you do on:	*Please judge how well this student does on:*
• Organization	• Organization
• Long-term projects	• Long-term projects
• Making a plan before starting work	• Making a plan before starting work
• Using strategies in my schoolwork	• Using strategies in his/her schoolwork
• Checking my work	• Checking his/her work
• Homework	• Homework
• Tests	• Tests
• Long-term projects	• Long-term projects

These examples reflect the discrepancies between students' self-perceptions and their teachers' judgments. In fact, students frequently overrate their level of academic performance in comparison with their teachers' ratings, as documented in many of our own studies and those of others (Meltzer et al., 2004a, 2004b; Stone & Conca, 1993; Stone & May, 2002). This discrepancy between teachers' and students' judgments is often linked with students' poor metacognitive awareness and with teachers' limited understanding of the extent to which executive function weaknesses are detrimental to students' performance.

When teachers understand these discrepancies and the reasons for them, they can use the MetaCOG questionnaires as a starting point for an important set of discussions with students and parents, so that they can all set common goals for the school year and can work toward these goals with similar expectations and objectives. Goal setting and prioritizing—two of the core executive function processes—can help students and teachers plan and reevaluate performance over the course of the school year (see Chapter 3).

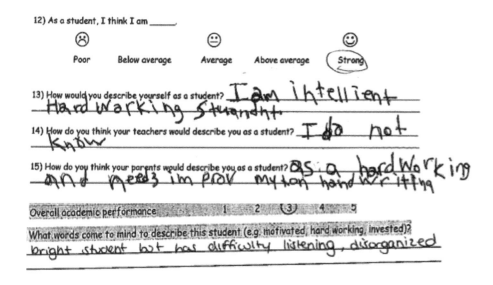

12) As a student, I think I am _____.

☹ Poor   😐 Below average   😐 Average   Above average   (☺ Strong) *if I try hard*

13) How would you describe yourself as a student? *I work hard and it is my goal to make it into M.I.T. or Harvard or get at least a decent masters degree.*

14) How do you think your teachers would describe you as a student? *academically strong but not great on effort.*

15) How do you think your parents would describe you as a student? *"You can be great if you try".*

Other comments: *I want to make the world (or "out there") a better place and I'm going to get the education to do it! School is great and it's very important when you grow up which I understand.*

Teacher Ratings and Comments:
Inconsistent effort, has trouble focusing; his work would be so much better if he could focus.

FIGURE 1.13a. Comparison of a student's versus a teacher's ratings of the student's school performance and effort.

12) As a student, I think I am _____.

☹ Poor   😐 Below average   😐 Average   Above average   (☺ Strong)

13) How would you describe yourself as a student? *I am intelligent Hard working stuandnt*

14) How do you think your teachers would describe you as a student? *I do not know*

15) How do you think your parents would describe you as a student? *as a hard working and needs im prov my ton hand writing*

Overall academic performance   1   2   (3)   4   5

What words come to mind to describe this student (e.g. motivated, hard working, invested)? *bright student but has difficulty listening, disorganized*

Teacher Ratings and Comments:
She is a bright student who has difficulty listening and is disorganized.

FIGURE 1.13b. Comparison of a student's versus a teacher's ratings of the student's school performance and effort.

HOW CAN TEACHERS ADDRESS THE NEEDS OF STUDENTS WITH EXECUTIVE FUNCTION WEAKNESSES?

> I could use the crazy phrases strategy for other things in school, because, you know, it's fun. Your mind is basically going to go for the fun stuff. . . . If it sounds like fun, it will help you remember more.
> —LEVON 11TH GRADER

Teachers can establish a strong foundation for executive function strategies when they teach their students to become metacognitive learners—that is, to think about *how* they think and learn. The questionnaire systems discussed above, such as the BRIEF and the MetaCOG, provide entry points for this process and help students to begin to reflect about the learning process and their specific learning styles. When instruction emphasizes metacognition and continually empowers students to use strategies, then students like Levon develop control over the learning process. As they begin to understand their learning profiles, they learn *when* to use strategies, as well as *which* strategies to use for *what* tasks. This self-awareness not only helps them understand their ongoing struggle to stay organized, but motivates them to learn and use executive function strategies for their academic work.

To meet the needs of students with executive function weaknesses such as Levon, a culture of strategy use should be created within every classroom and across the entire school. Teachers need to develop a systematic, strategic cycle of change that extends from school to home and back to school. When teachers stress that students' use of strategies is as important as accuracy, then strategy use becomes a habit of mind. This ensures continuity across the grades and generalization across content areas, so that students can understand and apply the strategies they learn on a continuing basis. Table 1.5 provides a few guidelines for creating a strategic classroom culture; more specific and detailed suggestions are given in Chapter 2.

Students' use of strategies occurs in stages, and they may initially use strategies incorrectly or unsuccessfully. For example, an early difficulty is reflected in

---

TABLE 1.5. How to Create a Classroom Culture That Promotes Executive Function

- Teach students to become *metacognitive learners* who think about *how* they think and learn.
- Make strategy use *count* by grading students on the basis of their use of strategies as well as their final answers.
- Use *strategy reflection sheets* for homework and tests, and give credit when students take the time to think about and explain *how* they have completed tasks.
- Strategy reflection sheets ensure that students allocate homework and study time to the processes as well as the strategies that work, rather than focusing on only the end product or content of learning.
- Create daily 5- to 10-minute *strategy-sharing discussions* for the class. These discussions are important opportunities for students to share their strategies with one another, as this process helps students to understand *how* they learn and think.
- Use *peer tutoring* to help students brainstorm with one another about whether or not an approach is an effective strategy for a specific task.
- Implement a *peer-mentoring* program to promote self-understanding, effort, persistence, and resilience in students with learning and attention difficulties.

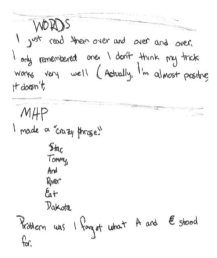

FIGURE 1.14. Self-reflection of Jay, a sixth grader, about the flaws in his approach to memorizing information such as lists of terms.

the comment of Jay, a sixth grader, that "I don't think my trick works very well" (see Figure 1.14). However, through self-reflection and self-regulation, students can eventually refine and apply these strategies to all the domains. Doing so will enable them to master more complex integrative tasks, such as writing, summarizing, note taking, and studying (Harris & Pressley, 1991).

HOW CAN CORE STRATEGIES BE TAUGHT ACROSS TASKS, CONTENT AREAS, AND GRADES?

> The way my mind works with that liquified gobble of dots, my notes would look scattered on a page. One of the most useful strategies I learned was three-column notes. With this system, I learned to make a hierarchy of notes and have it structure around itself and relate to things. This structure helped me to study and to write long papers.
> —BRANDON, COLLEGE GRADUATE

As noted above, students need to learn *when* to use *which* strategies and in *what* contexts. In particular, students need to recognize that not all strategies work for all tasks and all content areas all of the time. In other words, strategies need to be matched not only with the student's learning style, but with the task content and the context. Once students recognize the purpose and benefits of using strategies for tasks that are heavily dependent on executive function processes, they can be encouraged to personalize specific strategies, many of which can then be applied to different academic tasks across content areas and across the grades.

As Table 1.6 demonstrates, strategies in each of five selected executive function processes can be embedded in the curriculum at different grade levels. Students

TABLE 1.6. How to Scaffold Executive Function Strategies into the Curriculum across the Grades

Executive function strategies[a]	Common Classroom language: Grades 1–8	Metacognitive questions (for students to ask themselves)
Remembering/Acccessing working memory • Acronyms • Crazy phrases • Cartoons	Chunk Attach Meaning Rehearse	Can I review? Can I recite? Can I record? Can I picture it?
Organizing • Triple Note Tote • Mapping and webbing • Strategy cards	S²: Sort and Sequence or 4C's: Cluster, Categorize, Color, Chart	Can I sort into categories? Can I make a chart? Can I use color? Can I cut and paste the material?
Shifting • Shifty accents • Shifty images	"Let Go and Shift Gears"	Can I try another way? Can I make Plan A and Plan B?
Checking • Personal checklist • RE-view	"Top Three Hits" "Switch Pens"	What are my common mistakes? Did I switch pens?

[a]These strategies are all from BrainCogs (ResearchILD & FableVision, 2003).

can become metacognitive learners and can begin to understand when and where to use these strategies by asking themselves structured questions that help them to reflect.

Selected strategies that help students to organize, prioritize, and check can be taught in the first few grades in school and modified slightly for more complex tasks in the higher grades (see later chapters for more examples). For instance, the STAR strategy (see Figures 1.15a, 1.15b, and 1.15c) is a useful and very versatile strategy for summarizing reading material, organizing ideas for writing, taking notes, and studying in a variety of content areas (Meltzer et al., 2006). It helps students to plan, organize, prioritize, and shift between the main ideas and the details—whether they are reading for meaning or writing book reports in the first few grades (see Figure 1.15a), preparing complex science reports in the middle school grades (see Figure 1.15b), or completing challenging history assignments in the high school grades (see Figure 1.15c).

For essay writing or book reports, strategies like the STAR strategy can be used to help students focus on the major themes or main ideas. They can then use more detailed three-column note-taking systems to add relevant details to the paragraphs they write (e.g., the Triple Note Tote strategy from BrainCogs; see Chapter 2 for a fuller discussion). When all students—and particularly students with learning disabilities—use effective strategies such as these to develop their executive function processes, their academic performance often improves, which in turn enhances motivation and effort. This in turn results in more efficient and successful academic performance (Meltzer, 1996; Meltzer et al., 2001, 2004c), as

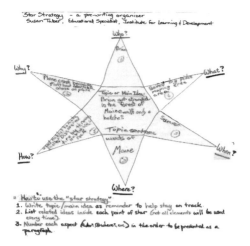

FIGURE 1.15a. The STAR strategy: An organizer for a fourth grader's book report about Hatchet by Gary Paulsen. From Meltzer and Krishnan (2007). Copyright 2007 by The Guilford Press. Reprinted by permission.

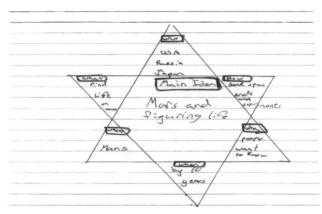

FIGURE 1.15b. The STAR strategy: An organizer for a seventh grader's science project about space travel to Mars. From Meltzer and Krishnan (2007). Copyright 2007 by The Guilford Press. Reprinted by permission.

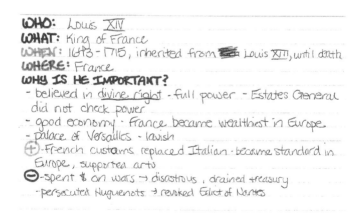

FIGURE 1.15c. The STAR strategy: An organizer for a 10th grader's history paper about the French Revolution.

described earlier. All these interconnected processes are essential for helping all students attain the academic success of which they are capable and deserving.

DRIVE TO THRIVE: A MODEL PROGRAM FOR INTEGRATING STRATEGIES INTO THE DAILY CLASSROOM ROUTINE

Drive to Thrive is a model program that integrates strategy instruction focused on executive function processes into the school curriculum (Meltzer et al., 2004b, 2007a; Meltzer, Sales Pollica, & Barzillai, 2007b; Noeder, 2007). The program creates a school and classroom culture where general and special education teachers have a shared understanding of the importance of nurturing efficient executive function strategies, focused effort, and positive academic self-perceptions in their students. *Drive to Thrive* incorporates the same philosophy as Graham and Harris's self-regulated strategy development (SRSD) (Graham & Harris, 2003; Harris & Graham, 1996; Reid & Lienemann, 2006), namely, that effective strategy instruction depends on student–teacher collaboration, and that strategies need to be personalized for each student, domain, and setting.

Within a *Drive to Thrive* classroom, classwork and homework focus consistently on the *how* of learning, rather than only on the final product. As a result, students begin to value the *process* of learning. Students are taught how to remember and recall previously learned information, and how to plan, organize and prioritize information for assignments and tests. There is an emphasis on flexibility and the ability to shift approaches in all learning and problem-solving situations. Independence is supported as students become increasingly aware of the benefits of using executive function strategies and are motivated to make the effort to continue using strategies that work for them. Over time, students begin to view themselves as capable learners; this results in positive mindsets and a willingness to make the effort needed to apply strategies to a wide array of tasks in different content areas.

Drive to Thrive focuses on building a cycle of academic success in all students through teacher training, use of multimedia software (BrainCogs), and peer tutoring (BrainCogs Squad). Participating teachers are trained to create a culture of strategy use in their classrooms, and to promote metacognitive awareness and strategy use in their students by embedding executive function strategies in their curriculum and daily teaching practices (see Chapters 2–7 for more detailed discussions). The following principles are emphasized (Meltzer et al., 2004a, 2004b, 2004c; Meltzer & Krishnan, 2007):

- Teachers foster metacognitive awareness and strategic mindsets in their students.
- Students and teachers view themselves as part of a community of learners who help each other to succeed and thrive.

- Students accept that hard work and focused effort are critically important for academic success, and that they will thrive if they have the drive.
- Teachers acknowledge that effort is domain-specific, and that students may sometimes need to work harder in one content area (e.g., math) than in another (e.g., language arts).
- Students recognize that persistence and determination are critically important for fostering academic and life success.
- Teachers gain an understanding of the close interactions among effort, strategy use, academic self-concept, and classroom performance, as well as the cycle that builds persistence, resilience, and long-term academic and life success.

In a series of 10 studies over the past decade, we have evaluated the efficacy of our *Drive to Thrive* program in six school systems with over 100 teachers and over 1,000 students (Meltzer et al., 2004a, 2004b, 2004c, 2006, 2007b). We have shown the importance of teaching strategies that strengthen the key executive function processes. We have also demonstrated that students' use of strategies in general and executive function strategies in particular, plays a critical role in school performance, and that it influences their perceptions of themselves as competent learners and good students (Meltzer et al., 2004b). For students with learning and attention problems, our findings have indicated that their self-perceptions often frame their willingness to work hard and to use strategies to compensate for or bypass their difficulties and to achieve greater success in school (Meltzer et al., 2004b). Students who develop an understanding of their learning styles, and of the importance of applying strategies to their schoolwork, begin to recognize that their struggles are not insurmountable. They also begin to recognize that they can be more successful academically when they learn and apply executive function strategies to their schoolwork (Meltzer, 2007; Meltzer et al., 2004b; 2007b; Noeder, 2007).

As displayed in Figure 1.16, our overall findings have shown that executive function strategies, in combination with effort, influenced students' performance on homework, and long-term projects, as well as their overall academic performance. It should be noted that R^2 refers to the amount of variability that can be explained by students' use of strategies as well as their effort.

Developmental differences, as well as shifts in the complexity of the school curriculum, frequently affect students' performance in ways that need to be understood by teachers and other school professionals (see Chapter 2 for more examples). In particular, changes in students' self-concepts and self-efficacy between the elementary grades (grades 3–5) and the middle and high school grades often affect their effort and academic performance. This is particularly evident in students with learning difficulties who are struggling academically. In one study of over 380 students, we identified changes between elementary and middle school that have important implications for the classroom (Meltzer et al., 2004b). In grades

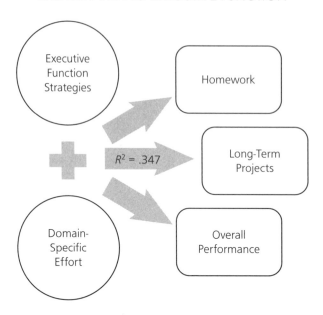

FIGURE 1.16. Combined effects of executive function strategies and domain-specific effort on academic performance.

3–5, regardless of whether students with learning difficulties judged themselves as good students or poor students, they still viewed themselves as hard workers who used strategies in their schoolwork (Meltzer et al., 2004b). They also judged themselves as working exceptionally hard in all academic areas—namely, reading, writing, spelling, math, science, and social studies. In contrast, at the middle school level, differences in academic self-concepts influenced students' judgments of themselves as good or poor students, as strategic learners, and as hard workers who were willing to make the effort to learn. Academic self-concepts particularly affected the effort and performance of students with learning difficulties: They were not as willing to work extremely hard in challenging academic areas that demand sustained effort and use of executive function strategies, such as writing, mathematics, science, social studies, homework, long-term projects, and studying for tests.

These findings have important implications for classroom teachers, given that written work, long-term projects, and assignments in content area subjects (e.g., science and history) often require students to write multiple drafts and exert maximal effort to revise, edit, and improve their work. Furthermore, as we have shown in our *Drive to Thrive* studies, successful strategy use mediates the relationship between students' self-reported levels of effort and their academic self-concepts (Meltzer et al., 2004a, 2004b, 2004c) and produces significant improvements in students' completion of homework and long-term projects, as well as in their overall academic performance.

CONCLUSIONS

The digital age has had a significant impact on the pace and efficiency of the workplace and there is greater demand for individuals who can solve problems efficiently and can develop and implement complex plans efficiently and accurately. As discussed in this chapter, because executive function processes have assumed increasing importance over the past decade, they need to be introduced into the classroom curriculum and taught systematically. Specifically, students need strategies for learning *how* to learn by shifting flexibly from the big picture (seen from the top of the mountain) to the numerous and often confusing details that need to be prioritized and organized (at the bottom of the mountain).

In the next six chapters, we discuss specific strategies that teachers can implement to help their students become successful learners who can master the challenges of 21st-century society, with its emphasis on executive function processes as well as rapid and efficient output. It should be emphasized that teachers are not expected to master all of the suggestions provided in this book, but rather to select those strategies and approaches that fit their own and their students' needs, and that can be integrated into the curriculum at appropriate times.

CHAPTER 2

Creating a Classroomwide Executive Function Culture That Fosters Strategy Use, Motivation, and Resilience

LYNN MELTZER and SURINA BASHO

> The students loved the strategies, and they all felt that they benefited from them. Students felt empowered, and I saw their skills become more internalized as they independently created their own organizational and memory strategies to study for their social studies and science tests.
>
> —FIFTH-GRADE TEACHER

Children become strategic learners when the schools they attend teach strategies explicitly and systematically, and require them to approach their classwork and homework strategically. A culture of strategy use in every classroom and across entire school systems ensures that students actively apply executive function strategies to all tasks. Within these types of classrooms, students experience themselves as important and valuable members of a community where they learn strategies from one another. When school systems and families foster the same values and emphasis on learning strategies, students' persistence, resilience, and academic success are promoted. Each child becomes part of an integrated classroom system, or a "child-in-classroom" (Bronfenbrenner, 1979; Doll, Zucker, & Brehm, 2004).

This chapter provides an overview of the key principles that are important for creating "strategic classrooms" and a classroomwide focus on executive function processes. We expand on the reasons *why* strategies that address executive function processes should be taught as part of the classroom curriculum. We then focus on *how* to create strategic classrooms by using key principles and approaches. Within this section, we also take a closer look at peer tutoring and peer mentoring in the classroom as ways of increasing students' motivation and engagement. Next, we discuss *what* specific executive function strategies can be embedded into content areas such as writing, reading, and math. We also provide a calendar that outlines strategy instruction focused on executive function processes across the school year. Finally, we discuss selected strategies that can be used to teach executive function processes within the context of writing, studying, and test taking.

WHY SHOULD INSTRUCTION IN EXECUTIVE FUNCTION STRATEGIES BE INTEGRATED INTO THE CLASSROOM CURRICULUM?

> When you go to class, even if you don't get the way the teacher's teaching, you might use strategies to turn it around and understand it your way, so you don't feel as dumb. Some kids, if they don't know that, they're just going to assume that they're dumb. They just might skip and not come to the class.
>
> —JOE, 11TH GRADER

As Joe's comments indicate, many students internalize their struggle with schoolwork as *"I'm not smart enough," "I feel dumb,"* or *"I'm just lazy."* Classroom teachers can empower students to take control of the learning process and to go beyond the "not smart" or "stupid" label by helping them to understand *how* they learn and *how* to apply strategies. In order to achieve this goal, teachers must ensure that strategies are systematic, consistent, and embedded in the classroom curriculum (Deshler et al., 2001; Hattie, Biggs, & Purdie, 1996). In other words, a "culture of strategy use" must be created in their classrooms (see Figure 2.1).

Over the past two decades, research has consistently indicated the importance of strategy instruction for enhancing students' conceptual understanding, their transfer and creative use of knowledge, and their ability to reflect on their own learning processes (Brown, 1997; Deshler, Schumaker, & Lenz, 1984; Pressley & Woloshyn, 1995). Studies have also shown that successful learners use effective strategies to process information (Brown & Campione, 1986; Harris & Gra-

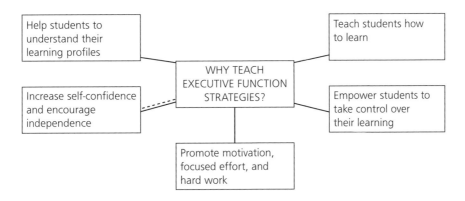

FIGURE 2.1. Why teach strategies that address executive function processes?

ham, 1992; Meltzer, 1993; Palincsar, Winn, David, Snyder, & Stevens, 1993; Pressley, Goodchild, Fleet, Zajchowski, & Evans, 1989). In fact, findings suggest that explicit instruction plays a critical role in helping all students to use metacognitive strategies to learn more easily (Deshler et al., 2001; Ellis, 1997; Harris & Graham, 1996; Graham & Harris, 2003; Meltzer et al., 2004a; Swanson, 1999; Zimmerman & Schunk, 2001).

Executive function strategies help students to go beyond the content that is being taught, so that learning is process-based rather than only outcome-based (Meltzer & Krishnan, 2007). Students need to learn *how* to set goals, plan, and prioritize; *how* to organize materials and information; *how* to remember and mentally recall previously learned information; *how* to "juggle" information in their minds; *how* to shift approaches in learning and problem-solving situations; and *how* to monitor themselves and check their work. All these executive function processes can be taught at all grade levels and applied to all content areas. For example, a strategy for writing a social studies report in the fourth grade can also be used for writing term papers in high school and college. In other words, although the content changes across the grades, the process or *how* of learning remains consistent across grade levels and content areas (Meltzer et al., 2006).

HOW CAN EXECUTIVE FUNCTION STRATEGIES BE TAUGHT IN THE CLASSROOM?

> Homework and tests are easier if you use more strategies. They help you see what types of things you need to work on a lot and what things you don't.
> —LESLIER, NINTH GRADER

As students develop an understanding of their strengths and weaknesses, as well as the demands of each learning situation, they realize the importance of executive function processes for academic success. When they use strategies that address the core executive function processes, they also become independent learners and flexible thinkers, and can more easily bypass their weaknesses while using their strengths to learn efficiently.

General Principles

Research on the implementation of strategy instruction has mostly focused on evaluations of students with learning disabilities in one-on-one and small remedial groups, rather than in general education classrooms (see Swanson & Hoskyn, 1998, for a review). Relatively few models exist for integrating strategy instruction systematically into the classroom environment. However, some classroom-based strategy instruction models and programs have emerged, such as the Kansas intervention model (Deshler, Ellis, & Lenz, 1996; Deshler & Schumaker, 1988), the

Benchmark model (Gaskins & Pressley, 2007; Pressley & Woloshyn, 1995), the SRSD model (Graham & Harris, 2003; Reid, 1996), the *Drive to Thrive* program (Meltzer et al., 2004c, 2007b; Meltzer & Krishnan, 2007; see Chapter 1), and the *SMARTS* (Success, Motivation, Awareness, Resilience, Talents, & Strategies) mentoring program (Gray, 2007; Gray, Meltzer, & Upton, 2008; Meltzer, 2007). Although each of these approaches includes a broad range of strategies and systems, a number of them address executive function processes. Several general principles for effective strategy instruction have been revealed through the use of these models/programs and are listed in Table 2.1.

More specific principles, important for creating a culture of strategy use in the classroom, are derived from our Research Institute for Learning and Development (ResearchILD) findings, as well as the meta-analysis of Swanson (1999). These principles include the following:

- Direct and explicit explanations of key concepts and vocabulary should be provided, so that students can access the information.
- The steps involved in learning specific strategies should be modeled.
- "Think-alouds" can be used to show students how to think about or approach a problem.
- Information should be broken down into manageable chunks or steps.
- Background information should be discussed to scaffold new concepts, so that all students have the same level of understanding.
- The goal of strategy use should be clear to both the teacher and the students (e.g., students should understand and apply at least one memory strategy independently on a test).
- Teachers should assess whether the goals are being met on a regular basis (e.g., track the number of times students spontaneously use a strategy in class).
- Teachers should assess whether students are using strategies effectively on a regular basis.

TABLE 2.1. Principles of Effective Strategy Instruction

- Strategy instruction should be directly linked with the curriculum.
- Strategies should be taught in a structured, systematic way, using scaffolding and modeling.
- Metacognitive awareness should be taught explicitly so that students develop an understanding of their profiles of strengths and weaknesses.
- Students' motivation and self-understanding should be addressed, to ensure that they generalize their use of strategies.
- Strategy instruction should address students' individual learning styles, motivation, and willingness to work hard—all critical for building the cycle of academic success.
- Hard work and effort should be encouraged and rewarded, as students initially need to work extremely hard to learn and use new strategies. Determination, persistence, and resilience are important, so that they do not feel overwhelmed by this initial effort.
- Time should be provided for practicing and applying strategies.
- Opportunities should be provided for students to extend and generalize strategies to a range of different tasks.

Day-to-Day Practice

When introducing a new strategy to students, it is essential to be systematic and to follow the general day-to-day practice guidelines outlined in Table 2.2. To ensure that students understand what, when, and how to use appropriate strategies, each teacher needs to create a classroom environment that is goal-oriented, fosters metacognition, and provides daily opportunities for students to use strategies to maximize their potential. The suggestions given in the next few pages provide a more detailed guide for teachers.

Set Goals for the Year, Month, Week, and Day

It is important for teachers to define explicit and measurable goals for strategy instruction. We recommend that teachers create overall goals for the year, as well as monthly, weekly, and daily goals. Setting goals provides a focus for instructional efforts and a framework within which to work. Consider these examples:

- *Goal for the year*: To ensure that each student in the class ends the year with at least five strategies he or she uses consistently. This should include one strategy from each of the five core executive function areas (i.e., planning, organizing, remembering, shifting, and self-checking).
- *Goal for the month*: To teach one organizational strategy each week.
- *Goal for the week*: To integrate a shifting strategy into the lesson plan.
- *Goal for the day*: To name and model specific strategies a few times over the course of the day.

One way for teachers to monitor whether they are meeting their goals in teaching executive function strategies is to use the Measure of Teacher Practice (MTP) questionnaire (Meltzer et al., 2007b). This questionnaire helps teachers reflect on and assess the extent to which they are teaching these strategies in the different academic areas. Figure 2.2 shows the application of the MTP to writing.

TABLE 2.2. Teaching Executive Function Strategies: General Guidelines for Day-to-Day Practice

1. Ensure that students understand what each strategy is.
2. Ensure that students understand what the strategy is used for.
3. Help students understand when to use the strategy.
4. Help students understand how to use the strategy.
5. Model the strategy for students.
6. Ask students to try using a specific strategy, either as a whole class, in pairs, or in small groups.
7. Have students reflect on how well the strategy worked for them as learners.

Measure of Teacher Practice (MTP)

Teacher: _____   Date: _____

Grade: _____

Please rate the extent to which you teach strategies systemarlcally when you teach writing. Please rate yourself on a 1–3 scale (1 = Seldom taught, 2 = Sometimes taught, 3 = Systematically taught).

Planning

Break down instruction and assignments into manageable steps.	1	2	3
Provide scaffolding for initiating writing assignments.	1	2	3

Organizing

Give explicit instruction about organization, relative to genre.	1	2	3
Provide graphic organizers, maps, and webs for teaching organization of ideas.	1	2	3

Prioritizing

Provide procedure checklists to prioritize important steps for the writing process.	1	2	3
Offer explicit instruction regarding key elements of writing.	1	2	3

Remembering/Juggling information mentally

Use mnemonics/crazy phrases to help students remember and juggle key steps in writing.	1	2	3
Encourage the use of strategies to help students to juggle information mentally.	1	2	3

Shifting

Provide instruction for varied vocabulary use and transition phrases.	1	2	3
Teach shifting strategies for multiple outcomes, audiences, and genres.	1	2	3

Self-checking

Use teacher- and student-made checklists for editing work.	1	2	3
Provide class time and direct instruction for revision of written work.	1	2	3

Please rate whether or not you include the following in your classroom instruction (0 = No, 1 = Yes).

Grading of written assignment includes credit for strategy use.	0	1
Visual reminders of strategy use are posted in the classroom.	0	1
Time is allocated for discussion of strategy use among students.	0	1
Time is allocated for students to reflect on personal strategy use.	0	1
Strategy use is personalized to students' academic needs and learning styles.	0	1

© Research ILD 2005

FIGURE 2.2. The Measure of Teacher Practice (MTP) in the writing area.

Establish a Starting Point for Tracking Progress

At the start of the school year, teachers will want to know each student's level of metacognitive awareness and strategy knowledge. A barometer reading can be taken of how much students know about strategies and what they think of themselves as learners. Teachers can develop their own questionnaires or can use the MetaCOG instruments discussed in Chapter 1 (Meltzer et al., 2001; Meltzer & Krishnan, 2007; Miller et al., 2001). As described there, the ME asks students to rate how hard they work and how well they do in selected academic areas, such as reading, writing, math, homework, studying for tests, and long-term projects. On the STRATUS, students are required to reflect on and to rate their use of strategies in the key executive function processes. Once teachers know where students are starting from, it is easier to evaluate and track the students' progress over time and then adjust the baseline to their learning needs. Teachers can also rate their students' effort and strategy use on the *TPSE* (again, see Chapter 1) and can compare their own ratings with their students' self-ratings on the ME. Establishing a baseline for understanding students' use of executive function strategies allows teachers to plan instruction more easily. This also helps teachers to determine the consistencies and inconsistencies between their own perceptions and those of their students. As Chapter 1 has shown (see Figure 1.5 there), students and their teachers often have very different perceptions of the students' performance.

Allow Adequate Time for Strategy Instruction in the Classroom

It takes time to teach students what executive function strategies are, why we use them, and what different types of strategies exist. As a result, it may feel as though strategy instruction takes too much time to implement in the classroom, compared to focusing only on the content. However, once the foundation has been laid for strategy instruction, less and less time is needed to integrate strategies into the curriculum. Furthermore, time is saved for teachers as students become more efficient, more accurate, and more effective. Consistency over time, as well as effort on both teachers' and students' parts, will ensure that strategy use becomes automatic. The approaches described below provide practical, easy-to-implement systems for making strategy use count in the classroom.

Foster Metacognition in Students

Teachers can make strategy use a required part of their curriculum by grading students on the processes and strategies they have used to reach their goals, in addition to the end product. The suggestions listed below provide practical, easy-to-implement systems for fostering metacognitive thinking in students and only involve a minimal amount of extra work for teachers.

STRATEGY REFLECTION SHEETS

Teachers can require students to use strategy reflection sheets for selected assignments, so that they gradually become accustomed to reflecting about *how* they learn and documenting their approaches informally (see the examples in Figures 2.3, 2.4a, and 2.4b). Each homework assignment or test should include a strategy reflection sheet at the end, for students to record the strategies they have used to complete assignments or to study for tests. When teachers count students' strategy use as part of the grade, the students begin to value the reflection process. It should be noted that teaching students to complete these strategy reflection sheets takes a little time, because it requires students to become metacognitive learners by thinking about *how* they think and learn.

As is evident from Figure 2.3, strategy reflection sheets can use a multiple-choice format, so that students do not have to rely on their expressive language skills to explain their thinking. Alternatively, students can be required to explain their thinking in more detail, using the open-ended format of the examples shown in Figures 2.4a and 2.4b.

STRATEGY NOTEBOOKS

All students can develop personalized notebooks in which they jot down the strategies that work best for them. These notebooks provide students with a place where they can easily store and refer to their favorite strategies, so that practice is made easier.

Drive to Thrive

Strategy Reflection Sheet

Check off the strategies you used to study for this test.

_____ Flash cards/Strategy cards   _____ Two-column notes

_____ Triple Note Tote (*BrainCogs*)   _____ Mapping/webbing

_____ Acronyms   _____ Discuss with a parent/friend

_____ Crazy Phrases (*BrainCogs*)   _____ STAR strategy

_____ Other _____

© Research ILD 2004

FIGURE 2.3. Strategy reflection sheet with multiple-choice format to scaffold and teach strategy use.

Date: 11/20/06
Subject: Writing Prompt

Drive to Thrive

Strategy Reflection Sheet

What strategies did you use to ~~study~~ prepare for this test or assignment?

Some strategies I used to prepare for this test were I used information that I already knew to think up a basic outline, and to fill in the gaps, I either used my notes, the textbook, or common sense.

© Research ILD 2006

FIGURE 2.4a. A sixth grader's strategy reflection sheet to assess strategy use for studying and taking tests.

Date: 11/20/06
Subject: writing prompt

Drive to Thrive

Strategy Reflection Sheet

What strategies did you use to ~~study~~ prepare for this test or assignment?

I used a graphic organizer plus all my notes that I had and a text book. Finally I use a little imagination.

© Research ILD 2006

FIGURE 2.4b. A fifth grader's strategy reflection sheet to assess strategy use for homework.

CHARTS AND GRAPHS OF STUDENT PERFORMANCE

To motivate students to use strategies, teachers can help students track their progress and strategy use by charting or graphing their performance on homework, tests, projects, and writing assignments.

PERSONALIZED ERROR CHECKLISTS

Students can also keep personalized checklists on their desks as reminders of the importance of checking strategies. These lists can include steps to check off before turning in a test, before finishing writing an essay, and before completing a math problem.

OTHER TECHNIQUES FOR ENCOURAGING STUDENTS' SELF-REFLECTIONS

Teachers can help students to access previous memories of success by asking leading questions, such as "Do you remember how easy the last vocabulary test was when you used a particular strategy? Why don't you try that again?" or "Do you remember the last time you made an outline before writing your essay? Wasn't it much easier to write when your ideas were organized?"

All these classroom techniques encourage students to reflect on how well each of the strategies has worked for them, and to review the strategies that best match their individual profiles of strengths and weaknesses.

Create a Strategic Classroom Environment

Students learn best when they gain knowledge through exploration, active learning, and visual imagery (Marzano, 2003). They need an opportunity to work through the process of experimenting and assessing the effectiveness of each strategy. They also need time in the classroom to learn and apply different executive function strategies. The following classroom-based systems help students to become metacognitive learners.

STRATEGY-OF-THE-WEEK DISPLAY BOARDS

Weekly classroom displays can be created to represent effective strategies used by students. At the start of each week, teachers can introduce a new strategy on the display board and can refer to this strategy throughout the lessons.

A STRATEGY WALL

One wall in the classroom can be dedicated to examples of students' use of executive function strategies. The key here is to make the strategies stand out in the

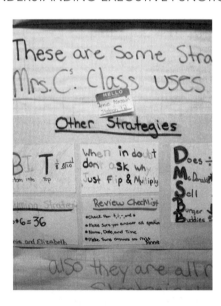

FIGURE 2.5. Example of a strategy wall in a fifth-grade classroom.

classroom, so that the students have daily visual reminders of effective strategies (see Figure 2.5).

STRATEGY-SHARING DISCUSSIONS

Teachers can create daily or weekly discussion times where students share their favorite personalized strategies from that week's classwork and homework. During these strategy-sharing discussions, students can teach other students their own strategies, and this process fosters metacognition and self-reflection. Teachers can also provide numerous examples of ways to apply strategies to everyday life (e.g., mnemonics for remembering a grocery list, crazy phrases for remembering the correct sequence for the months of the year, cartoons for remembering difficult vocabulary).

Practice, Practice, and More Practice!

STRATEGY PRACTICE LABS

Practice labs offer a chance for students to apply the different strategies they have been taught. With practice, the use of many strategies will become automatic, and students will also begin to recognize the efficacy of specific strategies for selected tasks. For example, one class period per week can be designated as strategy lab time, and students can experiment with a learning strategy that is useful for the content material.

MODELING STRATEGY USE THROUGHOUT THE SCHOOL DAY
AND ACROSS SUBJECT AREAS

Once students are able to assess which strategies work for them, they need to practice using the strategies with homework, classwork, and tests. For instance, teachers can create opportunities for students to use the vocabulary related to strategies by requiring that students:

- Discuss with each other how they can use specific strategies.
- Organize folders for different subjects.
- Practice making strategy notecards for new vocabulary.
- Practice using acronyms to remember important dates and events in history.

Make Strategy Use Count

As suggested earlier, strategy use should be included in the grading system across content areas. In other words, a small percentage of the grade should be assigned for students' use of selected strategies, and the remainder can focus on accuracy as well as content knowledge.

HOMEWORK

Homework assignments can include strategy reflection sheets or notecards, where students record the executive function strategies they use when they complete their reading, writing, or math homework, or when they study. For instance, instead of only writing down vocabulary words and their definitions, students could be required to select the five most difficult words and to create a memory strategy such as a Triple Note Tote card (see later discussion). In addition to using strategy reflection sheets or cards, students can be required to prepare a presentation about their favorite homework strategy. A grade can be assigned for how well each student explains the strategy and demonstrates how it works. For example, fifth graders who were involved in our *Drive to Thrive* study described their uses of strategies as follows:

- "I have a checklist for what I need to bring home with me."
- "I use Triple Note Tote to learn vocabulary and the colonies for social studies."
- "For social studies, I use crazy phrases before the test."
- "I use ANN E. BOA from BrainCogs."
- "I use webbing for the MCAS [Massachusetts Comprehensive Assessment System] open response."

EFFORT GRADES

An effort grade can be assigned to indicate how frequently students use strategies to prepare and study for their tests. This can also serve as a tracking system for teachers to document whether students' approaches to studying for tests change and improve over time.

TEST PREPARATION AND TEST-TAKING STRATEGIES

Strategies used to study and complete tests should receive additional credit. Students should be required to use strategies to answer selected questions on tests, and part of the grade should be assigned for their use of strategies.

Getting "Buy-In" from Students

One of the most important underpinnings of successful strategy instruction is to get "buy-in" from students, so that they feel invested in using appropriate strategies. A powerful approach is to show students how specific strategies can improve their performance. For instance, within the first week of school, students can be given a challenging test that requires the use of working memory strategies to do well. After the test, students can be taught a number of different memory strategies (e.g., the crazy phrases, acronyms, and cartoon strategies from BrainCogs). Students can be required to practice and use the strategies in class. When the teacher feels that students understand the memory strategies and can apply them, then the same test can be given again. After the teacher has scored the second test, students can review their scores on both tests, to compare their performance with and without the use of the memory strategies. Students will then have evidence of how strategies can improve their performance in school and on tests.

There are likely to be some students who feel they do not need strategies to help them in school because they already do well. It is important to help them understand that tasks will become more complex and challenging in high school and college, and that executive function strategies are essential for their continued academic success. All students—including high achievers, low achievers, and students with diagnosed learning and attention problems—need to learn strategies, particularly in the earlier grades, so that they can prepare for the fast pace and heavy organizational demands of academic work in the higher grades.

Strategy Group, Pair, Share

Strategy instruction should be provided in whole groups, small groups, and pairs. Just as teachers group students carefully for content area instruction, they also need to group students carefully for strategy instruction. Work on differentiated instruction (Tomlinson, 1999; Tomlinson, Brimijoin, & Narvaez, 2008) has shown that grouping students should be a dynamic process that depends on students' (1) content knowledge, (2) expertise, and (3) strategy preferences. In other words, students can be grouped together flexibly to learn a specific skill or strategy. These groups can be formed and disbanded for a variety of purposes. For instance, a student who is a second-language learner could be paired with a student who is a fluent speaker when the class practices using a specific strategy. The second-language learner then receives one-on-one support when practicing the strategy.

The Power of Peer Tutoring and Peer Mentoring

Peer mentoring and peer tutoring are powerful ways of teaching strategies and have significantly more positive effects on students' academic achievement, self-esteem, social competency, and peer relationships than teacher instruction alone (Mastropieri et al., 2001; Mastropieri & Scruggs, 2000). Furthermore, structured peer-tutoring programs have been shown to be extremely effective for students with and without learning difficulties (Fuchs, Fuchs, & Burish, 2000).

BrainCogs Squad is one example of an effective peer-tutoring system that is designed to facilitate strategy instruction in groups of students. It has been used effectively with middle school and high school students as part of ResearchILD's *Drive to Thrive* and *SMARTS* programs (Meltzer et al., 2007b). A BrainCogs Squad consists of approximately five to six students who are selected by the teacher to be peer tutors and are trained to navigate the BrainCogs software, apply the learning strategies, work with their peers, and assist teachers in using BrainCogs. BrainCogs is a multimedia system for teaching 13 strategies in the five key executive function areas (ResearchILD & FableVision, 2003) (see Figures 2.6a and 2.6b).

The BrainCogs Squad peer-tutoring system helps to create a bottom-up approach for teaching strategies that increases students' "buy-in," as well as their willingness to make the effort needed to use strategies in their classwork and homework. Each BrainCogs Squad peer tutor meets with five other students once a week for 1 hour to teach, review, and apply the selected strategy of the week. The 13 strategies are taught by the teacher and the BrainCogs Squad captains over the course of 13–26 weeks, depending on whether or not specific strategies need to be reviewed and practiced. Over these 13 weeks, the "buzz" created by the BrainCogs Squad in the class motivates students to learn and apply executive function strategies to their schoolwork, as the following comments by fifth graders in a *Drive to Thrive* classroom indicate:

"I like BrainCogs Squad because . . .
"The people that are teaching you may be your friends, and I think it's pretty cool."
"It's very helpful for studying."
"I understood the strategies better when my friend explained them to me."
"I could memorize something easily, using crazy phrases and cartoons."

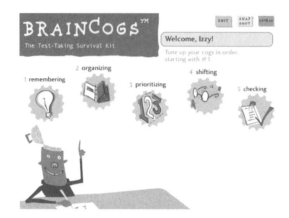

FIGURE 2.6a. The five executive function areas covered in BrainCogs. From ResearchILD and FableVision (2003). Copyright 2003 by ResearchILD and FableVision. Reprinted by permission of ResearchILD.

The Five Cogs

The five "cogs" in this CD-ROM represent different cognitive processes for learning and studying. There are 13 total strategies taught within the program, grouped according to the different cogs.

remembering

- Crazy phrases – make up a wacky sentence to help remember names, places, or events in a specific order.
- Acronyms - a real or nonsense word where each letter in the word is the first letter of something you're trying to remember.
- Cartoons – a picture you draw that helps you remember key information.

organizing

- Strategy cards – an index card with a question and a strategy for remembering the answer on one side, and the answer on the other.
- Triple Note Tote – a chart to use for taking notes from a textbook.
- Mapping & Webbing – a visual way to organize main ideas and supporting details.

prioritizing

- 1-2-3 Blastoff! – helps you relax, read carefully and begin a test.
- Red Flag – a mark to make on a test next to any question that's too hard to answer right away.
- ANN E. BOA – an acronym to help find seven tricky words on tests.

shifting

- Shifty Words – see more than one meaning in a word by shifting the accent or making nouns into verbs and vice versa.
- Shifty Images – find the meaning of a word by looking for clues in the surrounding words.

checking

- Your Personal Checklist – make a list of the usual mistakes you tend to make on a test.
- RE-view – how to change your focus at the end of a test so checking your answers is more successful.

FIGURE 2.6b. Thirteen strategies in five executive function areas can be effectively taught using a peer-tutoring model embedded in a strategic classroom culture. From ResearchILD and FableVision (2003). Copyright 2003 by ResearchILD and FableVision. Reprinted by permission of ResearchILD.

"When friends are teaching, it is way more laid back."

"You can learn new things about organizing things."

Similarly, the BrainCogs Squad captains who provide the peer tutoring feel empowered, as reflected in these comments:

"I like being a BrainCogs Squad peer tutor because . . . "

"I love all of it! Running the program is a lot of fun."

"I like being able to teach others."

"I like getting to help other people."

"Things get taught in a language kids can understand."

"It makes it easier because they're your friends, so you know how to work with them."

The BrainCogs Squad captains help to spark effort, motivation, and persistence among both themselves and their classmates. The peer-tutoring model increases student engagement, which in turn influences student motivation and achievement of classroom goals (Ryan & Deci, 2000). Furthermore, the BrainCogs Squad program turns the teaching and learning of strategies over to the students themselves. As a result, the students feel more invested in using these strategies and are willing to put forth more effort into learning, applying, and reviewing strategies. BrainCogs Squad has been an extremely successful component of the *Drive to Thrive* classrooms, and our research findings have demonstrated the sustainability of a classroom program that includes a peer-tutoring component focused on teaching executive function strategies (Meltzer et al., 2007a; Meltzer et al., 2010; Noeder, 2007).

Model Lesson Plans for Creating Strategic Classrooms

For teachers who plan their school year with a focus on creating a *Drive to Thrive* culture in their classrooms, it may be helpful to follow the broad time frame and series of lesson plans in Table 2.3. As this table shows, teachers can focus on each of the five executive function areas for approximately 2 months at a time. Teachers are encouraged to use this table as a guide and to teach these executive function processes flexibly on a continuing basis. A variety of techniques can be used, including software programs such as BrainCogs and Essay Express (ResearchILD & FableVision, 2005), which provide systematic and explicit presentations of strategies addressing the core executive function processes. In addition, teachers can scaffold the strategies and can require students to apply them to a range of tasks spanning nonacademic and academic areas. For instance, one idea is to have students plan and present a "strategy fair" at the end of the year, where they can creatively share with other classes what they have learned about executive function strategies.

TABLE 2.3. Timeline for Teaching Executive Function Strategies over the Course of One School Year

September to mid-October

Overview: Laying the foundation for strategy instruction

- *Barometer reading*: Establish where your students are in their understanding of strategies and metacognition (e.g. use the ME and STRATUS from the MetaCOG, as well as reflection sheets).

- *Create buy-in*: Give your students a challenging test at the beginning of the first week. A week later, after you have introduced and modeled a memory strategy, give students the same test and require them to use strategies to complete the test. Have them compare their "before" and "after" scores.

- *Introduce strategy language and define the following concepts and terms*: Strategies; executive function processes used in the classroom (e.g., organizing, prioritizing, memorizing, checking, shifting); metacognition; self-reflection.

- *Model strategies*: Explicitly model a few strategies for the students, to help them understand what they are.

- *Establish a strategic classroom*: This includes setting up strategy notebooks, a strategy board at the front of the classroom, a strategy wall, strategy reflection sheet routines, strategy-sharing discussions, and a BrainCogs Squad.

- *Student reflection*: Ask students to reflect on what they have learned. For instance, what terms did they have difficulty learning? Are there concepts they did not understand? What can they do to understand the concepts/terms better? Students should be asked to reflect on their learning consistently, to promote metacognition.

Mid-October to end of November

Overview: Memory strategies

- *Barometer reading*: Assess where your students are in their understanding of executive function strategies and metacognition (e.g., give them a test on the concepts and terms, and/or use reflection sheets).

- *Introduce and define memory strategies with an emphasis on working memory strategies*: Introduce crazy phrases, acronyms, and cartoons from the BrainCogs software, and/or use the memory strategies from Chapter 5.

- *Model memory strategies*: Explicitly model *what, when*, and *how* strategies can be used for retrieving information and mentally "juggling" details. Model for students how to be metacognitive learners by demonstrating (e.g., in a think-aloud) how to approach a problem and apply a strategy.

- *Active student learning*: Give students time in the classroom to learn the memory strategies and to apply them. Let them individually (or in dyads and groups) work through the process of exploring, experimenting, and assessing the effectiveness of each strategy.

- *Reinforce memory strategies*: Embed general and working memory strategies into lesson plans; use practice labs; require evidence of strategy use on homework/tests; have the BrainCogs Squad review and apply the selected strategy of the week with other students.

- *Student reflection*: Ask students to reflect on what they have learned. For instance, what memory strategy worked the best for them and why? For what kinds of problems could they use memory strategies?

- *Challenge students*: After your students have mastered the different strategies, challenge them to come up with their own strategies. That is, make them think critically about what works best for themselves as learners. Have the students share their original strategies with other students.

Beginning of December to mid-February

Overview: Organizing strategies

- *Barometer reading*: Assess where your students are in their understanding and use of general and working memory strategies (e.g., give them a test on the different types of memory strategies they learned and when/how to use them, and/or use reflection sheets). If you find that the students need more instruction and practice time with the strategies, then do not move on. Once you feel they understand the concepts and can apply them, then move forward.

(cont.)

TABLE 2.3. *(cont.)*

- *Introduce and define organization strategies*: For example, you can introduce strategy cards, Triple Note Tote, and mapping/webbing from the BrainCogs software, and/or use the organizing strategies from Chapter 4.
- *Model organizing strategies*: Explicitly model *what, when*, and *how* organizing strategies are used. Also model for students how to be metacognitive learners by demonstrating (e.g., in a think-aloud) how to approach a problem and apply a strategy.
- *Active student learning*: Give students time in the classroom to learn the organizing strategies and to apply them. Let them individually (or in dyads and groups) work through the process of exploring, experimenting, and assessing the effectiveness of each strategy.
- *Reinforce organizing strategies*: Embed organizing strategies into lesson plans (e.g., Triple Note Tote can be used for taking notes in class); use practice labs; require evidence of strategy use on homework/tests; have the BrainCogs Squad review and apply the selected strategy of the week with other students.
- *Student reflection*: Ask students to reflect on what they have learned. For instance, what organizing strategy worked the best for them and why? For what kinds of problems could they use organizing strategies?
- *Challenge students*: After your students have mastered the different strategies, challenge them to come up with their own strategies. That is, make them think critically about what works best for themselves as learners. Challenge the students to teach their strategy to other students or to the class. Then have a discussion about what worked and what didn't.

Mid-February to beginning of April

Overview: Prioritizing strategies

- *Barometer reading*: Assess where your students are in their understanding and use of organizing strategies (e.g., give them a test on the different types of organizing strategies they learned and when/how to use them, and/or use reflection sheets). If you find that the students need more instruction and practice time with the strategies, then give them more time before moving on.
- *Introduce and define prioritizing strategies*: For example, you can introduce 1-2-3 Blastoff!, Red Flag, and ANN E. BOA from the BrainCogs software, and/or use the prioritizing strategies from Chapter 3.
- *Model prioritizing strategies*: Explicitly model *what, when*, and *how* prioritizing strategies are used. Also model for students how to be a metacognitive learner by demonstrating (e.g., in a think-aloud) how to approach a problem and apply a strategy.
- *Active student learning*: Give students time in the classroom to learn the prioritizing strategies and to apply them. Let them individually (or in dyads and groups) work through the process of exploring, experimenting, and assessing the effectiveness of each strategy.
- *Reinforce prioritizing strategies*: Embed prioritizing strategies into lesson plans; use practice labs; require evidence of prioritizing strategy use on homework and tests; have the BrainCogs Squad review and apply the selected strategy of the week with other students.
- *Student reflection*: Ask students to reflect on what they have learned. For instance, what prioritizing strategy worked the best for them and why? For what kinds of problems could they use prioritizing strategies?
- *Challenge students*: After your students have mastered the different strategies, challenge them to come up with their own strategies. That is, make them think critically about what works best for themselves as learners. Challenge the students to teach their strategy to other students or to the class. Then have a discussion about what worked and what didn't.

Beginning of April to mid-May

Overview: Shifting and checking routines

- *Barometer reading*: Assess where your students are in their understanding and use of prioritizing strategies (e.g., give them a test on the different types of prioritizing strategies they learned and when/how to use them, and/or use reflection sheets). If you find that the students need more instruction and practice time with the strategies, then give them more time before moving on.
- *Introduce and define shifting and checking strategies*: For example, you can introduce shifty words, shifty images, personal checklists, and RE-view from the BrainCogs software, and/or use the shifting and checking strategies from Chapters 6 and 7.

(cont.)

TABLE 2.3. *(cont.)*

- *Model shifting and checking strategies*: Explicitly model *what, when*, and *how* shifting and checking strategies are used. Also model for students how to be a metacognitive learner by demonstrating (e.g., in a think-aloud) how to approach a problem and apply a strategy.

- *Active student learning*: Give students time in the classroom to learn the shifting and checking strategies and to apply them. Let them individually (or in dyads and groups) work through the process of exploring, experimenting, and assessing the effectiveness of each strategy.

- *Reinforce shifting and checking strategies*: Embed shifting and checking strategies into lesson plans; use practice labs; require evidence of shifting and/or checking strategy use on homework and tests; have the BrainCogs Squad review and apply the selected strategy of the week with other students.

- *Student reflection*: Ask students to reflect on what they have learned. For instance, what shifting or checking strategy worked the best for them and why? For what kinds of problems could they use shifting and checking strategies?

- *Challenge students*: After your students have mastered the different strategies, challenge them to come up with their own strategies. That is, make them think critically about what works best for themselves as learners. Challenge the students to teach their strategy to other students or to the class. Then have a discussion about what worked and what didn't.

Mid-May to June

Overview: Review of all strategies

- *Barometer reading*: Assess where your students are in their understanding and use of *all* the strategies (e.g., give them a test on the different types of strategies they learned and when/how to use them, and/or use reflection sheets). If you find that the students need more instruction and practice time with certain strategies, then provide classwide instruction as well as BrainCogs Squad peer instruction.

- *Strategy fair*: Your students can create a "strategy fair" where they display their favorite strategies and demonstrate their use to other classes in their school. This provides an incentive for the students to review the strategies they have learned over the past year.

- *Student reflection*: Ask students to reflect on what they have learned about strategies during the school year. As a class, you can discuss how to continue to use strategies the following school year, so that your students hold onto what they have learned.

WHAT EXECUTIVE FUNCTION STRATEGIES SHOULD BE EMBEDDED IN THE CURRICULUM ACROSS SUBJECT AND CONTENT AREAS?

> I learned very specific strategies that allowed me to succeed in school and in life today like multicolumn notes. These were a lifesaver for me. My notes would look scattered on a page. With this system, I made a hierarchy of information and had it structured around itself and I could relate it to things. . . . So if I had a history test I could think back to that note page and it all fitted into place—as opposed to remembering a liquefied gobble of notes that I had picked up here and there along the way.
> —BRANDON, COLLEGE GRADUATE

Reading comprehension, writing, math problem solving, summarizing, note taking, long-term projects, studying, and test taking all require students to integrate and organize multiple subprocesses simultaneously and to shift approaches on an ongoing basis. Success in all these academic areas is dependent on students' ability to make use of executive function processes in the five core areas. When strategies are embedded in the teaching of reading, writing, math, and content area material, it is possible to address these key executive function processes, as shown in Figure 2.7 and Table 2.4.

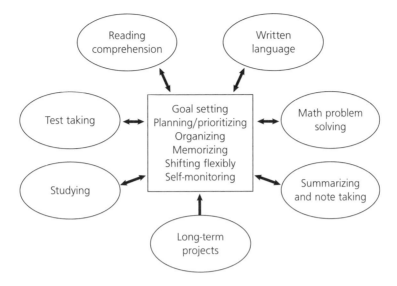

FIGURE 2.7. Core executive function processes that affect academic performance.

In the section below, we summarize a few of the strategies that can be used to teach writing, the basis for most academic work from the early grades into college. Because our 21st-century schools now emphasize strong writing skills as a requirement for academic success, we discuss strategies that can be incorporated into daily writing instruction as well as note taking, studying, and test taking. Teachers can use this discussion as guidance for strategy instruction in other academic areas (e.g., math, social studies, science). When these strategies are successfully incorporated into instruction, they increase the likelihood of future strategy use and academic success (Graham & Harris, 2003; Harris & Graham, 1996; Harris, Graham, & Mason, 2003; Meltzer et al., 2007b; Reid & Lienemann, 2006; Scardamalia & Bereiter, 1985; Zimmerman & Risemberg, 1997).

Writing

> I used BOTEC right now when I was doing my English test. I described
> it—Brainstorm, Organization, Thesis, Elaborate, Conclusion . . .—you know.
> Then I just attacked the thesis and examples first, and the rest just came.
> —LEVON, 11TH GRADER

Not only are writing skills heavily emphasized in today's schools, but standards-based tests, including the SAT, now incorporate a required writing section. As a result of this shift, students from late elementary school onward are frequently required to complete lengthy writing assignments, long-term projects, and essay tests that rely on executive function processes. Writing can be an overwhelming process for many students, because it requires the coordination and integration of a broad range of cognitive processes and skills, including memory, planning, generating text, and editing/revising their work (Flower et al., 1990; Flower, Wallace,

TABLE 2.4. Embedding Executive Function Processes and Strategies across Curriculum Areas

Curriculum area	Executive function processes involved	Strategies
Reading comprehension	Planning	• Use monthly calendars to plan and break down the reading of longer texts.
	Prioritizing	• Have students use active reading strategies that ask them to look for and mark specific aspects of the text (characters, setting, themes, etc.).
	Organizing	• Require students to use Post-it notes to summarize each chapter of a novel.
	Organizing	• Have students use story organizers to summarize stories for book reports.
	Shifting	• Have students predict different endings to a story.
Written language	Planning	• Require students to plan long-term writing assignments by using monthly and weekly calendars and setting short-term "due dates" for themselves.
	Prioritizing	• Have students use graphic organizers for brainstorming, prioritizing, and organizing ideas.
	Organizing	• Provide templates or specific guidelines for writing thesis statements, introductions, body paragraphs, and conclusions.
	Self-checking	• Help students develop personalized editing checklists based on previous assignments. Provide a specific rubric for students to check their work.
	Shifting	• Emphasize how to shift from the main ideas to supporting details when writing.
Studying and test taking	Planning	• Have students plan their study schedule for upcoming tests.
	Organizing	• Have students take notes from the textbook in a question–answer or Triple Note Tote format for later use as a study tool.
	Shifting	• Teach students to rephrase topic sentences as questions, and to use context clues to understand ambiguities and to interpret questions.
	Memorizing	• When requiring students to take notes and to study history or biology, teach them to develop their own acronyms or crazy phrases to help them to retrieve and manipulate the information.
	Self-checking	• Allow students to bring personalized checklists to tests, to remind them to check for their own common errors.

Norris, & Burnett, 1994). Many students also struggle to organize their ideas for writing, and they need the writing process to be broken down explicitly with organizers and templates that match both the goals of the assignment and their learning styles (Graham & Harris, 2003; Harris & Graham, 1996). They benefit when they are systematically taught strategies that address executive function processes (Bruning & Horn, 2000; MacArthur, Graham, & Fitzgerald, 2006; Ransdell & Levy, 1996; Zimmerman & Risemberg, 1997).

Writing templates and graphic organizers need to be explicitly structured in such a way that students can translate their ideas into paragraph form. These graphic organizers can be used successfully for different content areas and genres of writing, including book reports, persuasive essays, descriptive paragraphs, news articles, summaries, reflections, and narratives (Schunk & Swartz, 1993). Graphic organizers taught in middle school to help students plan and prioritize their ideas for essay writing can be extrapolated to more complex reports and papers at the high school and college levels (see Chapter 1). Rubrics like the one in Figure 2.8, from the *Drive to Thrive* program, can help teachers and students to analyze the writing process and embed executive function strategies in their teaching. For instance, the Figure 2.8 rubric can be used by teachers to explain, teach, and grade the writing process. In turn, students can use this type of rubric to provide structure when they are required to write a paper or complete an essay question on a test.

Students often struggle to break down the writing process into manageable components, and they benefit from strategies that help them to analyze, structure, and remember the steps involved. Strategies that provide such structure help students to plan, organize, prioritize, and check their work, so that writing a paper does not feel as overwhelming. BOTEC, a strategy from Essay Express (ResearchILD & FableVision, 2005), helps students to approach the writing process systematically through Brainstorming, Organizing, generating a Topic sentence (or Thesis), providing supportive Evidence (of Elaborating), and generating a Conclusion. Figure 2.9 illustrates a template for one part of the BOTEC strategy (marshaling evidence). When students experience success as a result of using a strategy such as BOTEC, they are more willing to apply the strategy to more complex writing assignments and projects.

As part of their writing assignments, students can also be required to complete and submit strategy reflection sheets. Strategy reflection sheets that incorporate structured questions and a multiple-choice format remind students of the range of strategies they can apply in producing and editing their written work (see Figure 2.10). When students understand the range of appropriate strategies, they can then be required to complete open-ended strategy reflection sheets (see Figure 2.11), which give them opportunities to use strategies creatively. Also, when they are given credit for using these strategies, they are more likely to make the effort needed to continue this process.

Note Taking, Studying, and Taking Tests

Summarizing, note taking, and studying are extremely challenging for students with learning difficulties, because all these tasks require the coordination and integration of multiple subskills and processes. On timed tasks, these students experience even more difficulty, and their performance often does not match their intellectual ability.

Strategies that help students to streamline and structure a large volume of information can make a significant difference in their performance. Strategies for organizing, prioritizing, and memorizing information are extremely important,

Drive to Thrive: Writing Rubric

Executive Function Processes	Below Average	Needs Improvement	Proficient	Exemplary Performance	Earned Points
Planning	**1 point** Little or no evidence of planning.	**2 points** A planning sheet is included, but it is incomplete.	**3 points** Student includes an outline or graphic organizer that is partially filled out. Planner is somewhat related to final essay.	**4 points** Student includes completely filled-out outline or graphic organizer, and final essay reflects its use.	
Organizing	**1 point** Student does not include a rough draft.	**2 points** Student includes a partially completed rough draft that does not follow an organizational plan.	**3 points** Student includes a rough draft that roughly follows his/her outline or graphic organizer.	**4 points** Student includes a rough draft that is well organized and follows the planning tool.	
Shifting	**1 point** Student shows no changes from the rough draft to the final draft.	**2 points** Only slight evidence of improvement is seen between the rough and final drafts.	**3 points** Student makes at least two changes beyond spelling and punctuation in the final draft.	**4 points** The student takes a different point of view in the final draft, or makes at least three major improvements between the rough draft and the final draft.	
Prioritizing	**1 point** Essay includes no transition words to show sequence, contrast, or relative importance of ideas.	**2 points** Essay includes only transition words, such as "and," "also," and "but."	**3 points** Essay includes two more sophisticated transition words that indicate sequence, importance, or contrast, such as "however," "on the other hand," "another example," etc.	**4 points** Essay includes more than two transition words to connect ideas or paragraphs.	
Checking	**1 point** Student does not submit a checklist with the writing project.	**2 points** Student checks for a few mistakes but not for others.	**3 points** Student checks off the checklist to indicate that he/she checked most of the items on the list.	**4 points** Student submits checklist indicating that he/she has checked for each item on the list. Student's writing reflects no errors that are listed on the checklist.	
				Score:	

FIGURE 2.8. Writing rubric from the *Drive to Thrive* program. Adapted from Meltzer, Sales Pollica, and Barzillai (2007b). Copyright 2007 by The Guilford Press. Adapted by permission.

Brainstorm
Organize
Topic Sentence
Evidence
Conclusion

EVIDENCE:
Idea #1: Being tired
    Detail not enough sleep
    Detail long school day

Idea #2: More important things
    Detail Jobs
    Detail activities

Idea #3: Understands
    Detail not paying attention
    Detail being bored

CONCLUSION:
People have obstacles that affect students.

FIGURE 2.9. A ninth grader in the *SMARTS* program uses the BOTEC strategy to organize evidence for a project presentation about reducing the homework load in school. The template is from ResearchILD and FableVision (2005). Copyright 2005 by ResearchILD and FableVision. Reprinted by permission of ResearchILD.

Strategy Reflection Sheet

What strategies did you use for this writing assignment?

_____ BOTEC   _____ Personalized checklist

_____ Mapping and webbing   _____ Sentence starters

_____ Graphic organizer   _____ Introduction template

_____ Linear outline   _____ Other

© ResearchILD 2004

FIGURE 2.10. Strategy reflection sheet for writing: Structured questions that scaffold the writing process.

Strategy Reflection Sheet

What strategies did you use for this writing assignment?

_____

_____

© ResearchILD 2004

FIGURE 2.11. Strategy reflection sheet for writing: Open-ended questions.

as these reduce the load on working memory and improve efficiency as well as accuracy.

In this section, we briefly summarize a few strategies that are particularly useful for a wide range of academic tasks; Chapters 3–7 describe specific strategies for each of the five executive function areas in greater detail. Graphic organizers and three-column note-taking systems help students to organize and memorize information simultaneously. One example is the Triple Note Tote strategy (from Brain-Cogs; ResearchILD & FableVision, 2003), which can be used for taking notes, summarizing, and memorizing information in content areas such as key terms or new vocabulary. In all cases, the major concept is written in the first column, important details in the second column, and a paired visual–verbal strategy for remembering the information in the third column (see Figures 2.12a and 2.12b).

Students also benefit from memory strategies such as mnemonics and crazy phrases for organizing information, reducing the memory load, and retrieving information for tests or projects. For example, when students are required to study the states and their capitals for a test, crazy phrases and personalized diagrams help them to chunk the information for easier recall (see Chapter 5 for more specific examples). Finally, personalized error checklists help students to edit and correct their written work during homework and tests. Once students analyze their most common errors, they can develop a checklist and an acronym to help them to remember the items on the list, so they can check their work independently. Although general checklists work for many students, personalized checklists help students to be aware of and search for their own most common errors (Dunlap & Dunlap, 1989). One student may consistently make spelling errors but may have no difficulty with organization; another may have the opposite profile. Figure 2.13 illustrates a personalized checking strategy developed by a fifth grader who used a crazy phrase and acronym to remember his most frequent errors and the details he needed to check. Personalized checklists like this one are useful for all students, whether or not they have difficulty completing their homework accurately, make careless errors on tests, have difficulty with the mechanics of writing, or struggle to remember the steps in a math problem.

CONCLUSION

When schools build an executive function culture across classrooms, they empower students to learn *how* to learn and *how* to solve problems flexibly—processes that are critically important for success in the global world we now live in. When schools and families foster the same emphasis on learning strategies, persistence and a strong work ethic are promoted, and these should lead to academic and life success. As students learn effective approaches to their work, their motivation, self-confidence, and resilience also increase.

Definitions

Term	Definition	Example/Strategy
River Basin	An area of land drained by a river and its tributaries often surrounded by land of higher elevation	Amazon basin
Peninsula	A narrow strip of land surrounded on 3 sides by water	
Isthmus	A narrow strip of land connecting 2 larger pieces of land	Isthmus of Panama
Elevation	height of the land	*elevator*
River source	the start of a river usually in the highlands	START
River mouth	the place where the river flows into a larger body of water	
Plateau	a flat land at high elevation	*plateau*
Plain	an area of level land usually at low elevation and often covered by grasses	

FIGURE 2.12a. Triple Note Tote strategy from BrainCogs. The template is from ResearchILD and FableVision (2003). Copyright 2003 by ResearchILD and FableVision. Reprinted by permission of ResearchILD.

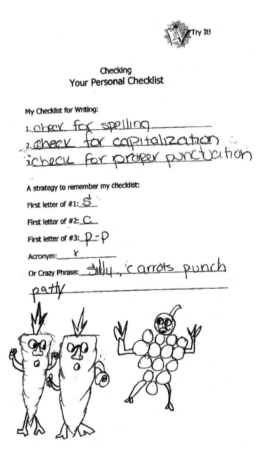

Triple Note Tote and Cartoon:

TRIPLE NOTE TOTE FOR BASIC ALGEBRAIC TERMS

Term	Meaning	Strategy for remembering
Line Segments	beginny end	The book has a beginny and a end
Rays	Has a begining Point and no end	Ray of Sun — The sun is attacking

FIGURE 2.12b. Triple Note Tote strategy from BrainCogs. The template is from ResearchILD and FableVision (2003). Copyright 2003 by ResearchILD and FableVision. Reprinted by permission of ResearchILD.

Try It!

Checking Your Personal Checklist

My Checklist for Writing:

1. check for spelling
2. check for capitalization
3. check for proper punctuation

A strategy to remember my checklist:

First letter of #1: S

First letter of #2: C

First letter of #3: P=P

Acronym: x

Or Crazy Phrase: silly carrots punch patty

FIGURE 2.13. A fifth grader's personalized checklist for writing. The checklist itself is from ResearchILD and FableVision (2003). Copyright 2003 by ResearchILD and FableVision. Reprinted by permission of ResearchILD.

PART II

SCAFFOLDING EXECUTIVE FUNCTION
PROCESSES INTO THE CURRICULUM CONTENT

CHAPTER 3

Goal Setting, Planning, and Prioritizing

The Foundations of Effective Learning

Kalyani Krishnan, Melissa J. Feller, and Melissa Orkin

In life, goal setting, planning, and prioritizing are critically important for the successful accomplishment of a wide range of activities. Similarly, in the classroom, a student's ability to set goals, manage time, plan, and prioritize lays the foundation for success. In this chapter, we discuss the executive function processes involved in goal setting, planning, and prioritizing and suggest strategies for supporting and fostering the development of these processes in classrooms and across grades.

WHY SHOULD WE TEACH STRATEGIES FOR GOAL SETTING, PLANNING, AND PRIORITIZING?

Executive function processes pose a unique challenge to educators because of their complex nature. Specific processes such as goal setting and planning are implicit in many of the tasks assigned to students from elementary school onwards. For instance, a third grader who was asked to complete a book report was provided with directions by her teacher as shown in Figure 3.1. In order to complete this task, this third grader needed to set both long-range and short-term goals (i.e., "I need to finish the book report before Halloween and do my best" as a long-term goal, and "I need to read 25 pages every day" as a short-term goal). In order to reach her goals, this student needed to plan her time and to allocate an appropri-

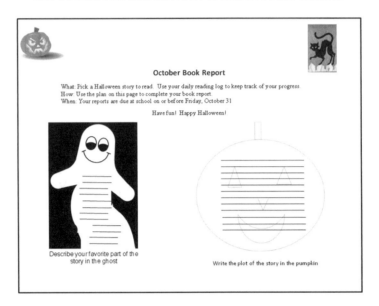

October Book Report

What: Pick a Halloween story to read. Use your daily reading log to keep track of your progress.
How: Use the plan on this page to complete your book report.
When: Your reports are due at school on or before Friday, October 31

Have fun! Happy Halloween!

Describe your favorite part of the story in the ghost

Write the plot of the story in the pumpkin

FIGURE 3.1. Sample third-grade book report assignment.

ate amount of work to each day. Finally, the student needed to prioritize multiple matters. Of all the books in the library, which one would she choose? Of all the ideas in the book, which one was the most important to include in the summary? Of all the funny and interesting things that happened in the story, which one was her favorite?

Thus what appeared to be a simple third-grade project was in fact a multilayered challenge that required this student to use several executive function processes, such as setting goals, planning tasks, and developing priorities in an independent manner. This, along with other such projects that are assigned to children of all ages, provides a powerful rationale for explicitly teaching specific strategies for these processes to children throughout the grades. We devote the first half of this chapter to goal setting, and the second half to planning and prioritizing.

WHY SHOULD WE TEACH EXPLICIT STRATEGIES FOR GOAL SETTING?

Goal setting refers to the learner's ability to identify a guiding purpose for his or her actions, based on an awareness of personal strengths and limitations and a clear vision of the desired final result (Locke, 1968). In order to meet a goal, the student needs to carefully organize his or her approach, both by taking into account the "big picture" and by recognizing the smaller steps involved (see Chapters 1 and 2). Timely and successful execution of tasks also relies on the ability to plan and prioritize.

In the classroom, there is a need to strike a balance between a curriculum-centered view of education and a student-centered view. Typically, the curriculum is predetermined, and the teacher's job is to deliver the content to the students. Thus it is the teacher's job to set the goals and objectives for each lesson, to determine the pace and direction of each lesson, and to mediate the learning experiences of students in a very direct manner. However, as discussed in Chapters 1 and 2, recent changes in education have led to the inclusion of more long-term projects and research papers across the grades, all of which require more independent engagement from students. As a result, teachers need to share the goal-setting process with students, to help the students to become independent learners. The importance of teaching goal-setting strategies is supported by research findings that show a strong cyclical relationship between the ability to set personal goals and sustain higher levels of motivation on the one hand, and the development of positive self-efficacy (which promotes success) on the other (Pintrich & Schunk, 1996; Schunk, 1995). Research evidence also suggests that students may be more energized and interested when they engage in tasks of their choosing, and that they may work harder on self-made goals than they do when they work toward the plans and expectations of others (Linskie, 1977). Our clinical experience suggests that when teachers share the goal-setting process with students and give them appropriate guidance, students can learn how to set reasonable goals, which increases their motivation and willingness to persist.

Although most educators begin to think about goal setting as a desired learning outcome in secondary school and when they are planning for students' transitions to postsecondary education, research has shown that children at much younger ages can set specific and meaningful goals that influence their learning outcomes (Fuchs, Fuchs, & Deno, 1985; Johnson, Graham, & Harris, 1997; Licht, 1983; Missiuna, Pollock, & Law, 2004; Missiuna, Pollock, Law, Walter, & Cavey, 2007). In fact, when children learn to set effective personal goals, and when their learning is supported by meaningful feedback (self-assessment and teacher feedback) as well as by appropriate learning experiences and strategies, they show improvements in their academic performance. For example, given a complex process such as writing, research suggests that children are more easily able to manage the multiple demands of the task when they learn how to self-regulate their efforts through goal setting and planning (De La Paz, 2007; Graham, 2006). Research evidence also shows that this is true both for typically developing children and for students with learning challenges (Carlson, Booth, Shin, & Canu, 2002). Indeed, while all students benefit from learning how to set goals, students who struggle with academic tasks benefit even more.

Thus there are compelling pedagogical reasons for teaching students how to set goals and for making goal setting an integral part of the classroom learning experience, beginning in the early elementary grades. In fact, goal setting needs to be taught explicitly, systematically, and across grade levels and curriculum areas

(Meltzer, 2007). However, given the pace of the curriculum, the diversity of learning styles represented in the classroom, and the large volume of content, many teachers find it difficult to make the time to teach goal setting, as it is not a component of the content-centered curriculum. Therefore, practical and manageable systems and strategies for embedding goal setting into the curriculum are discussed below.

WHAT FOUNDATIONAL PROCESSES ARE NEEDED FOR SUCCESSFUL GOAL SETTING?

In order to set effective and reasonable goals to guide their learning, students need to:

- Develop an understanding of their learning profiles.
- Understand the "big picture" or gestalt, and envision the endpoint of a task.
- Value the task or assignment.
- Learn to set goals that are proximal, specific, and appropriately difficult.

Self-Understanding

Self-knowledge and self-understanding are key essential metacognitive processes for goal setting. Many students with learning and attention difficulties demonstrate weaknesses in their self-knowledge and self-awareness, as well as in their strategy use and their self-efficacy (Stone & Conca, 1993; Swanson, 1989; Torgesen, 1977). Research has shown a strong cyclical relationship among self-understanding, effective strategy use, academic success, the development of beliefs that one can succeed, positive self-concept, and increased engagement with learning (Licht, 1993; Meltzer et al., 2004; Meltzer & Krishnan, 2007). Thus students who know that they learn best when they draw diagrams and visualize information are more likely to use these types of strategies when studying. Students who realize that it is difficult to remember math formulae are more likely to seek out appropriate memory strategies for studying. Therefore, students who are strategic are likely to experience academic success as a result of their proactive and engaged style, which in turn increases their self-efficacy (belief that they will succeed at a task). When approaching tasks from this position of strength, students can also become more engaged with challenging tasks and accept more responsibility for their own learning. In addition, when students self-evaluate their learning, this process also informs their teachers, who can align their classroom practices with the needs of their students (see Chapters 1 and 2; see also Joseph, 2003). Conversely, students who are not self-aware and introspective about their learning, and those who lack effective strategies, are at a great disadvantage when coping with the fast-paced and complex curriculum of today's schools.

Understanding the "Big Picture"

Awareness of the "big picture," and the ability to see it, are important factors that help students to set goals and plan a course of action (see Chapter 1). When students are focused on proceeding from one detail to the next, they often do not have a sense of the final product or goal (Meltzer, 2004, 2007; see Chapter 1). Thus they have a limited ability to take charge of their own learning. Many students with learning and attention difficulties tend to use a sequential, piecemeal approach to learning. Such an approach is tedious and may overload them with many details; at the same time, they lack an understanding of how these details fit together (Stein & Krishnan, 2007). On the other hand, students who are able to move flexibly back and forth between an understanding of a whole task and of its parts, or from "the top of the mountain to the bottom and back" (see Chapter 1), are better able to manage the complex, multilayered tasks typically required of students in our 21st-century schools. A related skill is the ability to envision the endpoint or final step in a process. When students can do this, they have a clear and well-defined target, which helps them to focus their effort and to allocate their cognitive resources effectively.

Valuing the Task

For students to engage actively with a task or assignment, it is important that they value this task. According to *expectancy–value theory*, individual expectations of success, combined with the value attributed to the goal, influence each student's level of motivation (Fishbein & Ajzen, 1975); see Figure 3.2. Therefore, a child who has a strong expectation of success and values a task will engage with it. If the child either does not expect success or does not value the goal, the child's motivation will be significantly compromised. Thus teachers need to ensure that students value the tasks they are asked to engage with, so that they will set meaningful and motivating goals (Adelman & Taylor, 1993; Deci & Ryan, 1985; Stipek, 1998).

> $E \times V = M$
> (the $\times$ represents a multiplication sign)
>
> In other words:
> Expectation of success $\times$ Value of the goal = Motivation

FIGURE 3.2. Expectancy–value theory diagram.

Setting Proximal, Specific, and Appropriately Challenging Goals

Students need instruction focused on how to set goals that are proximal, specific, and appropriately challenging (Harris & Graham, 1996). Research has shown that *proximal* goals—ones that will be accomplished in the near future, and therefore provide immediate incentives—are more effective than long-range goals in promoting student success (Schunk, 1980). For example, a proximal goal such as "I want to finish reading Chapter 3 today" provides a better incentive than "I have to finish reading this novel by the end of the month." Similarly, specific goals (e.g., "Make sure all your sentences start with capitals and end with periods") are more effective than vague goals (e.g., "Do your best!") on various types of tasks (Locke, 1968; Locke, Shaw, Saari, & Latham, 1981). Finally, the difficulty of a goal is often related to student engagement (Locke, 1968; Locke et al., 1981). However, the relationship between goal difficulty and student engagement can be complex. due to a student's temperament, self-efficacy, and other factors. Some students are motivated by harder goals, and they are willing to persist and exert great effort in order to succeed. Other students may doubt their ability to achieve a goal, may perceive it as "too difficult," and thus may not engage with the task. Therefore, while it is important to set increasingly challenging goals in order for students to progress, teachers need to take care that these goals are identified with an understanding of each student's capacity, as well as his or her tolerance for stress.

HOW SHOULD STRATEGIES FOR GOAL SETTING BE TAUGHT?

We can teach students to set goals through classroom accommodations and direct, systematic instruction.

Accommodations

Many common instructional accommodations provide students with scaffolds that help them with goal setting. Although these accommodations are often prescribed for students with learning or attention difficulties, they constitute "best practices" in general education. They include the following:

• *Rubrics and samples of finished projects* give students an opportunity to "look inside the teacher's mind." They help students to envision the endpoint, as discussed above, and make the task requirements explicit for all students. Providing both rubrics *and* samples also addresses the needs of students with multiple learning styles, including learners who prefer visual, verbal, part-to-whole, and gestalt-based (i.e., top-down) approaches.

• *Visual representations* (i.e., pictorial or three-dimensional) often clarify the ambiguities inherent in verbal descriptions (Bransford & Johnson, 1973). Teachers can use projects completed by previous students (photographs or actual examples), or can lead them through a sample prior to giving students a similar assignment. Many teachers in the lower elementary grades do this as a matter of routine, but these supports are less common in middle school and beyond. Older students continue to benefit from access to samples of completed projects, as well as from rubrics. When a students are given a comprehensive rubric, they have a clear idea of what the teacher is looking for and how performance may be assessed. A sample rubric for evaluating a student debate is provided in Figure 3.3.

• *The use of calendars and phased timelines* also promotes effective goal setting. Calendars provide visual reminders of due dates, as well as schemas for setting and achieving short-term goals that contribute to the successful attainment of the larger, final goal. A sample calendar is presented in Figure 3.4. Teachers and students can use several Internet sources to customize calendars. The Scholastic website offers the option to generate and customize a calendar that can then be printed out and kept in a student's binder (*www.scholastic.com/kids/homework/calendar.htm*). Another website that allows students and teachers several options is Calendars That Work, where a variety of calendar styles can be selected and printed so that students can manually fill in their deadlines and schedules (*www.calendarsthatwork. com*). Calendars and timelines are discussed in further detail later in this chapter.

Category	4	3	2	1
Respect for Other Team	All statements, body language, and responses were respectful and were in appropriate language.	Statements and responses were respectfu l and used appropriate language, but once or twice body language was not.	Most statements and responses were respectful and in appropriate language, but there was one sarcastic remark.	Statements, responses, and/ or body language were consistently not respectful.
Information	All information presented in the debate was clear, accurate, and thorough.	Most information presented in the debate was clear, accurate, and thorough.	Most information presented in the debate was clear and accurate, but was not usually thorough.	Information had several inaccuracies or was usually not clear.
Use of Facts/ Statistics	Every major point was well supported with several relevant facts, statistics, and/ or examples.	Every major point was adequately supported with relevant facts, statistics, and/or examples.	Every major point was supported with facts, statistics, and/ or examples, but the relevance of some was Questionable.	Not every point was supported.
Rebuttal	All counterarguments were accurate, relevant, and strong.	Most counterarguments were accurate, relevant, and strong.	Most counterarguments were accurate and relevant, but several were weak.	Counterarguments were not accurate and/or relevant.

FIGURE 3.3. Sample rubric for evaluating a student debate, created with an online template (*rubistar.4teachers.org/index.php*). Template used by courtesy of ALTEC at the University of Kansas.

Monday	Tuesday	Wednesday	Thursday	Friday
March 22 Think about people to inteview	23	24 Have the name of a person	25 Begin developing questions in class	26 Make contact by today and set up interview
29 Interviews begin Types questions due	30	31	April 1	2 →
5 Interviews continue —	6	7	8 →	9 All interviews done
12 Noes from inteviews due Make outline in class	13 Write oral history —	14	15	16 →
19 Rough draft due	20 Work on final draft and — illustration	21	22	23 →

Final draft and illustrations due on **April 26, 2010**

FIGURE 3.4. Sample calendar.

Direct and Systematic Instruction

In addition to the types of accommodations discussed above, all students benefit from explicitly learning how to set goals. Self-understanding, grasp of the "big picture," and valuing the task are among the key components of effective goal setting, as discussed above.

Self-Understanding

Promoting self-knowledge is a key factor in helping students become effective goal setters. Self-knowledge is an important component of a resilient learning style, which in turns ensures that students set reasonable and appropriate goals (see Chapters 1 and 2). When students receive formal evaluations, their profiles of strengths and weaknesses are clearly defined as a result of the testing. However, it is possible for all learners to reflect on their own learning and arrive at reasonable conclusions about their own strengths and weaknesses, whether or not they receive complex evaluations. There are several activities and surveys that class-room teachers can use to initiate discussions about learning styles. One effective way is to use a *multiple-intelligences wheel*, based on Howard Gardner's theory of multiple intelligences (Gardner, 1983). This can be adapted to the ages and ability levels of specific students. Teachers and students can color in different sectors to illustrate their own patterns of strengths and weaknesses. A sample wheel repre-senting a fifth grader's profile is shown in Figure 3.5.

Self-assessments are most effectively completed in a nonjudgmental environ-ment that is accepting of all learning styles. It is essential for teachers to begin creating such an environment by introducing students to the notion that everyone has different strengths and weaknesses. Given the widespread use of social skills programs such as Open Circle (a "social and emotional learning program" from the Wellesley Center for Women at Wellesley College; see Chapter 8), many stu-dents in elementary schools are familiar with inclusive discussions. These types of discussions help students to develop a rich and well-integrated understanding of their learning styles.

Teachers can complete an initial discussion and survey of different types of learning styles at the beginning of the year. Following this, it is important to con-tinue these discussions periodically throughout the year, so that all learners will continue to update their self-assessments. It is often helpful to use outstanding public figures to illustrate different learning styles, so that students can identify with acknowledged leaders. Once the stage has been set, teachers can capitalize on their students' developing self-awareness by promoting a classroom culture that welcomes multiple learning styles.

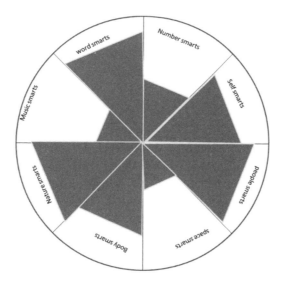

FIGURE 3.5. Fifth grader's multiple-intelligences wheel.

Understanding the "Big Picture"

Teachers can further facilitate goal setting by sharing the "big picture," or schema, with respect to broad goals for the year or the term, along with more specific content- or lesson-related goals. (A more in-depth discussion of schemas is presented in Chapter 4.) Understanding the broad sweep of the content they will be learning allows students to set their own personal goals more effectively. This also helps them to understand the relationship between the information that they already know and the new content that will be presented; doing so gives them a framework into which they can integrate their new knowledge (Stein & Krishnan, 2007). For instance, it is appropriate for a teacher to make the following types of broad statements at the beginning of the year. A statement to second or third graders regarding the goals or the science curriculum may be as follows:

> "This year, we are going to learn about the environment around us and how it affects living things. We will study weather, natural resources, and problems like pollution, and understand how plants, animals, and people adapt to their surroundings."

A possible statement to students in an advanced high school level English course may be this:

> "An essential component of this course is the development of proficiency in the language arts. The guiding principles of Advanced English II are as follows:
>
> - Speak and write clear, idiomatic English.
> - Engage in the writing process, from prewriting to editing and peer feedback to revision.
> - Develop voice and depth in both personal and literary papers.
> - Develop confidence, independence, and critical judgment relative to your own work.
> - Understand as fully as possible what is read."

Once these goals are articulated and discussed with students, they can set their own personal goals for the class in question, keeping in mind their own strengths and weaknesses, their personal interests, and the stated intent of their teachers. A blank Individual Goal Plan is provided in Appendix 1. A plan such as this can be tailored to meet the "good goal" requirements of proximity, specificity, and difficulty. Teachers and students can further customize these templates to meet their individual needs.

In addition to these broad, curriculum-related goals, students benefit greatly when their teachers "set the stage" as a new unit is introduced or when new concepts are encountered in an ongoing lesson. Teachers can use a variety of approaches to connect information as they teach and present a bird's-eye view of the organization of content. Diagrams, maps, and timelines, for instance, provide anchoring organizational frameworks in the humanities.

Teachers can also use graphics and organizational tools to synthesize and summarize the key concepts in a curriculum (see Figure 3.6). For instance, many students in grades 6–8 are introduced to the major early civilizations, with the overarching goal of helping them understand the underlying themes and patterns that were the governing principles for the establishment of human civilization. Although this is one of the stated goals for middle school social studies curricula, this information is rarely provided to students in a concise manner. Instead, students often study several ancient civilizations in sequence (e.g., Babylon, Egypt, Indus Valley), but they are left to abstract and synthesize key concepts independently. Students with executive function difficulties often struggle with these implicit curriculum goals. In contrast, when the teacher uses an organizer like the one shown in Figure 3.6, the information is encapsulated for all students so that they can understand the goals and intentions of the course as well as the way information is connected within this subject. Such an approach meets the needs of students with weak executive function processes in particular. This type of synthesis has the added benefit of promoting greater understanding and recall of key concepts in the humanities and sciences.

Other opportunities to set conceptual goals are provided by strategies such as K-W-L, which is used during reading activities (Bos & Vaughn, 2002). The K, W, and L stand for "what I <u>K</u>now," "what I <u>W</u>ant to learn," and "what I did <u>L</u>earn," respectively. By activating students' background knowledge and helping them set goals, this strategy promotes better reading comprehension. Similarly, during

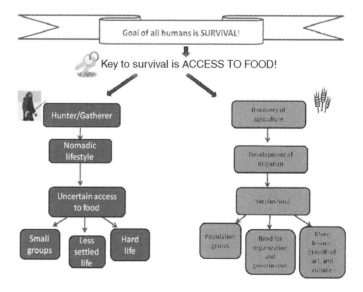

FIGURE 3.6. Bird's-eye view of curriculum content.

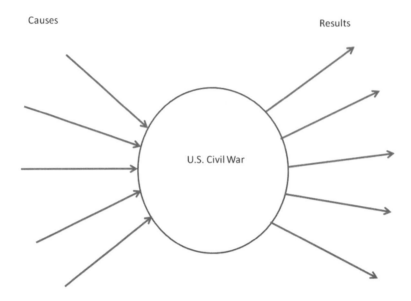

FIGURE 3.7. Template for generating a graphic summary: Causes and effects of the U.S. Civil War.

math problem solving, the practice of estimating an answer to a problem prior to computation is in fact a goal-setting task, whereby students try to limit the parameters of the outcome of their calculations.

Teachers can also use graphic organizers, including tools such as Thinking Maps (*www.thinkingmaps.com*), to establish the big picture and demonstrate the connections between different concepts within a unit. This information can be presented before, during, and after the lesson, and can play an important role in helping students synthesize and summarize information. For example, these types of strategies can be used at the conclusion of units as ways of recalling, integrating, and summarizing key points. The class as a whole can contribute to the summary as the teacher develops it on the board or overhead projector. The example provided in Figure 3.7 shows a template that can be used to generate a graphic summary of the causes and effects of the U.S. Civil War.

Valuing the Task

"How can I get my students to care about what I'm teaching?" This is a burning question for many teachers. Teachers are often frustrated with their students' lack of connection to the subject materials, especially at the upper grades. In order to solve this problem effectively, it is essential to understand that individuals are motivated to achieve goals that are in line with their own strong desires and values (Eccles, 1987; Feather, 1988; Vroom, 1964; Wigfield & Eccles, 2000). As White (1959) asserted, individuals have a deep-rooted desire to have an effect on their environment and to obtain results that they value within their own contexts. Furthermore, *self-determination theory* suggests that people are motivated to act in a manner that is consistent with their values (Deci & Ryan, 2000). These are powerful drives that exist in all learners.

Traditionally, teachers and parents have assumed that all students in the classroom are inherently motivated to learn. In years gone by, students who did not "fit" into traditional classrooms could achieve their goals through alternate routes, such as apprenticeships to various practical trades. More recently, life success is increasingly dependent on strong performance in secondary school, as well as prolonged engagement with formal learning through college and graduate school. As a result, there is an urgently felt need to engage all learners within the classroom, including those who have attention and learning difficulties as well as weak executive function processes. Teachers can harness students' drive to learn by helping all students value the work they do. To do this, in addition to including the above-discussed practices in their approaches, teachers need to show that *they* value specific strategies by doing the following:

• *Prioritizing highly valued strategies in the curriculum and agenda.* Teachers need to put the strategies they themselves value at the top of their "to-do" list, to make sure students know how much they are valued.

• *Providing sufficient time for students to learn and practice these strategies.* When teachers state expectations but do not allow time for students to apply strategies to meet these expectations, students get the message that this is not really important after all. Thus teachers need to "build in" time to teach, practice, and use the specific strategies in the classroom.

• *Making it count.* As discussed in Chapters 1 and 2, teachers need to hold students accountable and provide incentives for students to use strategies that are valued in the classroom.

Students can learn to value tasks by doing the following:

• Understanding how each specific skill or strategy can help them achieve a goal they value. An Individual Goal-Planning Worksheet is provided in Appendix 2. This worksheet helps students connect short-term objectives to long-term goals.

• Reflecting on their subjective experience of using a specific strategy and evaluating the impact this strategy has on their ability to succeed with tasks they value. For example, students who discover that setting goals helps them succeed in meeting deadlines may value this process more readily.

• Hearing from their peers about what *they* value in a specific strategy. Peer mentoring and peer opinions are excellent motivators for many students, particularly during adolescence (see Chapter 2 for a discussion of the BrainCogs Squad peer-tutoring approach).

As students master these goal-setting strategies, they simultaneously learn organizational strategies, all of which help them to succeed with multistep, open-ended assignments in today's classrooms. These organizational strategies are essential for keeping up with the quickening pace and larger volume of material covered in each advancing grade.

WHY IS IT IMPORTANT TO TEACH EXPLICIT STRATEGIES FOR PLANNING AND PRIORITIZING?

Planning and prioritizing are essential for success in today's classrooms. Each time students are asked, "What did you like best in this story?", "What were the main causes for this historical event?", or "What is the most important information in this math problem?", they need to prioritize information. The current emphasis on long-term projects and the expectations for independent homework completion even at the earliest grades have increased the demands on all students for independent planning and prioritizing. Thus students' ability to arrange tasks in order of importance and to use strategies for timely completion of tasks are directly related to their success and ability to achieve their goals across academic areas. Many teachers devote time to helping their students identify what is important by developing and providing study guides, teaching methods for identifying major themes in literature, or formulating theses for research papers. However, planning and prioritizing strategies also need to be taught explicitly and directly in regard to time and task management in general.

Effective planning and prioritization lead to efficient time management, which in turn has been found to increase productivity, alleviate stress, and have a positive effect on students' learning and achievement (Misra & McKean, 2000). Students who implement time management strategies are often considered to be more self-regulated, more aware of their thinking processes, and more able to manage their learning across contexts than those who procrastinate (Wolters, 2003). Perhaps this is because the facility to structure one's time, generate an accurate plan for project completion, and prioritize tasks also results in a greater likelihood of goal achievement and academic success.

Efficient time management is a combination of inherent abilities and learned strategies. However, the challenges of time management have become increasingly complex. Environmental demands, such as daily schedules packed with activities or "timeless" distractions like video games and social networking sites (e.g., Facebook and MySpace), can easily reduce a student's task efficiency and productivity. An added challenge lies in the fact that students rarely have control over their own schedules, as many of them rely on their teachers and parents to manage their time. Thus many students struggle to plan their time independently and break down tasks into manageable "bits" when pressured by deadlines. Just as students benefit from learning isolated decoding skills first and then practicing them embedded in context, mastering time management strategies in isolation before applying them in the context of fast-paced and complex curricula is critical. In fact, each component of the complex process of time management can be developed through the use of effective strategies that are practiced and reinforced in the classroom.

WHAT FOUNDATIONAL PROCESSES ARE NECESSARY FOR PLANNING AND PRIORITIZING?

Time management involves interactions among several different executive function processes, including goal setting, prioritizing goals, planning goal achievement, and prioritizing tasks to accomplish objectives (Britton & Tesser, 1991). These processes are fairly complex even for older students; therefore, it is important to begin by focusing on the foundational processes involved in time management:

- Knowledge of time
- Knowledge of task
- Prioritizing tasks
- Monitoring progress

Accurate Knowledge of Time

Understanding the passage of time is often referred to as "having a sense of time." However, unlike the basic five senses, which are innately developed, awareness of time relies on memory to provide cues for future predictions. For example, when trying to guess how long it has been since one has last had something to eat, one might consider all the events that have taken place between the last meal and the present time. If the events included a walk and watching a television program, one might estimate that a few hours had elapsed. However, if no TV program was watched, the estimate might be reduced by an hour. Estimating time is therefore a subjective process rather than an exact science, and a number of factors affect the precision of these estimates. For example, when students are bored, time tends to drag on; when they are actively engaged, time passes quickly. An individual's emotional state can also cause time to be either over- or underestimated. It is important that students learn to identify the factors leading to over- or underestimations of time, and that they are offered regular opportunities to hone their estimation skills. Overall, an accurate understanding of time provides a strong foundation from which students can begin to predict how different activities will fit into their schedules.

Accurate Knowledge of Tasks

Once students possess a sufficient understanding of time, they can move on to estimating the length of time they should allot for given tasks. Perfecting the ability to estimate a task is a stepwise process that improves with practice. It is first necessary to *divide* large-scale projects into small, manageable parts. Next, it is important to accurately *predict* the length of time it will take to complete each part. The final step in task estimation is perhaps the most important: Incorporating feedback to create a *revised* and more accurate estimate is critical for improving future predictions.

A student's precision in predicting the duration of an activity depends on that student's memories of previous experiences. When children are trying to predict how long it will take to make a peanut butter and jelly sandwich, they will have to think back to the last time they made that type of sandwich. It will also be necessary to consider all of the steps involved, from gathering supplies to spreading the toppings. They will have to check to see whether they have all of the needed supplies—and what happens if they have limited experience with sandwich making? How will this affect their predictions? Children with limited knowledge about an activity are likely to underestimate the amount of time needed to complete the task. However, if they break the task down into smaller, sequential steps, there is a stronger likelihood that accurate estimation will occur, even in the face of an unfamiliar task. Adults and children alike often underestimate the amount of time a task will take (Buehler, Griffin, & MacDonald, 1997; Josephs & Hahn, 1995). Therefore, children should be encouraged to overestimate the time needed to complete an unfamiliar task. If they do complete the task in less time, this will allow them to relax between activities.

Prioritizing Tasks

After students have estimated the amount of time to devote to each task, they will need to prepare a schedule and arrange the order in which the tasks should be completed. Prioritizing requires an understanding of each task and the role it plays in larger assignments. A student should learn to place tasks into three different categories—*obligation, aspiration,* or *negotiation*—based on their importance, time sensitivity, and role in the student's life.

- *Obligation.* These activities are mandatory tasks that are time-sensitive, such as homework, jobs, and chores. For some students, enrichment activities like soccer or violin practice also fall into the obligation category.
- *Aspiration.* These activities are enjoyable tasks that are interesting and important but are not obligatory. These types of activities usually include attending a friend's birthday party, going to a concert, or watching a favorite television program.
- *Negotiation.* These activities do not have immediate time constraints and are flexible (e.g., putting together a model robot). These activities are not as critical as either obligatory or aspirational tasks.

Categorizing activities is an important part of the prioritization process, because it provides a foundation on which students can build their schedules.

Once tasks have been grouped according to their importance, students can rely on their knowledge of time and task to allot the appropriate amount of time for each activity. Obligatory tasks should always be accommodated first, followed by tasks in the aspiration category. In order to ensure accuracy, the process of categorizing activities should involve input from multiple parties, including parents and teachers.

Monitoring Progress

Perhaps the most important skill under the time management umbrella is the ability to monitor progress. Students who are monitoring their progress should engage in such tactics as rearranging a schedule, identifying inefficient behaviors, and delegating or deleting responsibilities based on progress.

- *Rearranging schedules.* If students have a good working knowledge of time, familiarity with the task at hand, and the ability to determine the importance of completing the given activity within a short period of time, then they should be able to rearrange their schedules in light of unexpected occurrences. However, this type of flexible thinking can be the most challenging aspect of time management for many students. Rigid behavioral patterns may be due to inexperience with situations in which a student is solely responsible for planning his or her time. Alternatively, perhaps the student is accustomed to renouncing his or her plan, rather than reallocating time and resources once a schedule disruption occurs.
- *Identifying overcommitments.* When students are feeling stressed, they should be given an opportunity to identify a situation in which they have overcommitted themselves. The negative outcomes of an overcommitted schedule include emotional responses such as frustration or disappointment, as well as behavioral responses such as exhaustion, confusion, and outbursts. In order to avoid situations of overextension, students can be introduced to the processes of *delegation* and *deletion*. *Delegating* an activity involves asking another qualified individual to complete a task (e.g., asking siblings to complete chores and giving them a portion of an allowance, or asking a cocaptain to lead swim practice and offering to cover one of his or her team obligations in the future). For younger students, it may be necessary to identify that the act of delegating is appropriate in situations where important tasks need to be accomplished but a student is already overwhelmed. *Deleting* an activity from a student's schedule is only appropriate when the activity is not considered an obligation and would not result in undesirable consequences if neglected.
- *Reflecting on current time management strategies.* Opportunities to reflect offer students a chance not only to recognize when they have overextended themselves, but also to identify circumstances in which they have not performed at their optimum level because of inefficient time management strategies. Most educators have found that there is a strong correlation between incomplete or poorly executed work and the amount of time a student has allocated for completion. Students who

can reflect upon how their strategies for organizing and prioritizing time affect their outcomes will be better equipped to make effective use of time management strategies. For example, a student who receives an unsatisfactory grade on a large social studies project will undoubtedly feel disappointed. However, if that student can identify specific organizational behaviors that led to poor outcomes (e.g., saving work for the last minute), he or she will be one step closer to creating a more efficient plan for the future.

HOW SHOULD STRATEGIES BE TAUGHT FOR PLANNING AND PRIORITIZING?

Classrooms in which time management strategies are explicitly modeled and scaffolded by teachers, and then practiced independently by students, can help students become more organized and less stressed. This can be done at all grade levels by skillfully combining these elements:

- Explicit strategy instruction
- Systematic reduction of teacher support
- Making the expectation clear that assignments should be planned and organized, rather than simply completed, by students

Teaching Strategies to Promote Accurate Estimation of Time

Most students can improve their sense of time when teachers provide them with opportunities to practice estimating the passage of time in a neutral state, so that they are not stressed by the demands of larger projects or activities.

Elementary School

During elementary school, the majority of teachers present their students with highly structured schedules. Most early elementary educators not only post the daily activities for their students to follow, but also take responsibility for ensuring that transitions from one activity to happen smoothly. As a result, although they are operating within a highly structured environment, students are not necessarily provided with an opportunity to understand the mechanisms that underlie the ability to schedule effectively. By making an effort to highlight the strategies that contribute to time estimation, and providing students with opportunities for repeated practice, teachers will assist students in building their time management abilities.

- *Discussing the daily schedule.* Previewing the daily schedule not only provides students with the security of knowing what is to come, but also gives them a sense of how time can be divided. Expanding on the preview, teachers can discuss the timely features of tasks on the schedule. Activities can be qualified by their length, and compared to a predetermined list of similar-length activities. Perhaps spelling is a long activity like playing a soccer game, while lunch is a short activity like taking a bath. Making explicit connections between various activities in the students' lives will assist them in developing estimation abilities.

• *Providing visual representations.* Because time is an abstract concept, concrete visual and physical representations will assist younger students in their development of time estimation skills. Placing visual cues, dividers, or color-coded sections on clocks will provide tangible representations of the amounts of time remaining for given tasks.

• *Practice in monitoring time usage.* Classrooms that display a daily schedule not only provide students with a visual representation of structure, but also offer opportunities for students to become involved in time management activities. Students can take turns being the *time monitor* for different activities. The monitor, who can wear a clock around his or her neck or carry a timer, is in charge of providing 5-minute warnings and alerting the class about the conclusion of an activity.

Middle School

By middle school, students have typically developed a sense of time and can often independently and accurately estimate the amount of time to allot for simple, straightforward tasks. Yet, as their schedules become more demanding and their schoolwork increases in complexity, older students are likely to benefit from support in time estimation.

• *Further practice in time estimation.* Although middle school students are more adept than younger learners at estimating time for short activities, once distractions are present or a task increases in length, estimation can become a challenge. Incorporating estimation games like "Guess When a Minute Is Up!" (Figure 3.8) into class time can effectively illustrate the limits of our own estimation abilities and the importance of relying on estimation aids like timers and alarms.

• *Identifying individual strategies.* Once students have been made aware of their natural weaknesses in estimation abilities, they should be encouraged to identify the timing aids that best suit their needs. The Time Estimation Worksheet (Appendix 3) will help students to recognize the impact of distractions and their own limitations in tracking the passage of time. A collection of timers in a classroom will provide multiple means of assistance. Egg timers and alarms are perhaps the most widely used tools for tracking time; however, clocks are particularly helpful as well, as they illustrate both spatially and numerically how much time has passed. As students engage in classroom work, teachers can provide a variety of timing devices to choose from and can emphasize the importance of handing in completed assignments on time without prompting.

1. Begin by covering all the clocks in the room. Then ask students to sit quietly and then place their hands in the air when a minute has passed.

2. Record their times, and discuss the strategies they used to estimate time. Perhaps some students count, while others sing a quick song—all helpful techniques for estimating time.

3. Now ask the students to repeat the activity, but this time instead of sitting quietly, students should talk to their neighbors. Remind them during the activity to raise their hands when a minute has passed.

4. Record their times again and note the differences. Have students discuss ways in which the activity changed their ability to gauge time, and whether the minute seemed to pass more quickly or more slowly.

5. Discuss the reasons why this might be the case. This type of activity can be practiced regularly by covering all the clocks and incrementally increasing the amount of time that students must estimate (e.g., 3 minutes, 5 minutes, 7 minutes).

FIGURE 3.8. "Guess When a Minute Is Up!"

High School

High school students typically make independent choices regarding the order in which they will tackle their tasks and the ways in which they will schedule their time. Although they have usually established routines, high school students often do not reflect on the efficiency of their habits. Teachers can support the ongoing development of accurate estimation abilities by providing structured reflection opportunities following assignments.

Teaching Strategies to Promote Accurate Allotment of Time to Tasks

For students to allot adequate time to complex projects, studying for tests, or even accomplishing everyday tasks (e.g., walking the dog before school), they need to learn strategies for doing so. Perfecting the ability to estimate the time required for a task is a stepwise process that improves with practice and age.

Elementary School

During the primary grades, the daily schedule—often posted prominently in the classroom—is a wonderful platform for practicing task time estimation. Teachers can begin modeling such estimation for students by first breaking down tasks into smaller parts and then posting a task's estimated length on the daily schedule. Next, students can take on the role of *scheduler*.

• *Student schedulers.* During the beginning of the year, teachers usually establish and maintain the class agenda. By discussing the nature of each task on the schedule, breaking down more complex activities into component parts, and providing time estimates for each component and the total task, teachers model these strategies for the students. As the year progresses, students can take turns acting as the *scheduler* and filling in estimated times for each of the daily activities. When the students become more adept at estimation, the schedulers can take more responsibility and manage such challenges as revising estimates and rearranging activities.

Middle and High School

As assignments increase in difficulty and the volume of long-term projects intensifies, students should be provided with further opportunities to practice their task time estimation abilities. Middle and high school students who are familiar with accurate estimation strategies are more likely to demonstrate their knowledge successfully even in the face of complex, multicomponent assignments.

  • *Divide and conquer.* In order to become an accurate task time estimator, it is necessary to first *divide* a large-scale project into its smaller components, and then to *estimate* the length of time each part will take to complete. For example, conducting a science experiment on plant growth entails multiple steps. First, each step in the process needs to be identified; its length should then be approximated; and finally, the total duration of the project can be estimated. Figure 3.9 is a sample worksheet for breaking a large project down into smaller parts, tracking progress, and making revisions, which will aid in future task predictions.
  • *How long will it take?* In their daily schedules, students are likely to encounter many activities that require breaking a task down into multiple steps and estimating the length of time to allot to each step. For example, cooking dinner requires skillful task and time estimation in order to get multiple components of a meal on

Project Breakdown Worksheet				
Assignment Name	**Big Parts**	**Details**	**Predicted Time**	**Actual Time**
Essay on themes in <u>To Killa Mockingbird</u>	Reading the book (total 300 pages)	1–100	2 hours	3 hours
		100–200	2 hours	3 hours
		200–300	2 hours	3 hours
	Writing the essay	Taking notes	2 hours	1 hour
		Actual writing	4 hours	6 hours
		Editing	1 hour	1 hour
			15 hours/ 5 nights	17 hours/ 6 nights

FIGURE 3.9. Sample worksheet for breaking down a large project.

the table at the same time. Activities that facilitate the rehearsal of such skills can be easily incorporated into the classroom.

Teachers should select a fun activity that students are likely to encounter in their daily experience, such as making a sandwich. Working individually or in pairs, the students should break down the activity into smaller tasks. A food-related activity works well because it can naturally be structured like a recipe, including gathering ingredients and listing the steps (see Figure 3.10); however, a similar "Recipe for Success" format can be used with an academic assignment such as cleaning up after a science experiment (see Figure 3.11). The students should be asked to predict how long each individual step will take, as well as the total length of the activity.

Next, the students should pass their "recipe" to their neighbors, and the neighbors should then follow to execute the activity while keeping track of time. Afterward, the students should be encouraged to discuss their estimates and the consequences resulting from underestimating the actual time needed for completion (e.g., not being able to eat a completed sandwich). This worksheet can be modified and applied to many tasks, including the end-of-the-day packup, transitions between classes via the students' lockers, and so on.

Recipe for Success

Title
Jam Slam Sandwich

Ingredients or materials	
2 pieces of bread	Bananas
Jam	Granola

Steps
This is how I make it:
1. Get a plate, spoon, banana pieces, and granola.
2. Take two pieces of bread out of the bag.
3. Put two spoonfuls of jam on one slice of bread and spread the jam with the back of the spoon.
4. Use the spoon to put six pieces of banana on the bread.
5. Use the spoon to sprinkle granola on the bread.
6. Put the plain piece of bread on top of the other piece.

Steps	Estimated time	Actual time
Step 1		
Step 2		
Step 3		
Step 4		
Step 5		
Step 6		
Total		

Did I miss any steps?

FIGURE 3.10. Worksheet for the Recipe for Success activity, using an actual recipe.

Recipe for Success

Title	Ingredients or materials
Pack up and roll out of the lab	Cleaning supplies

Steps			
Steps 1. Turn off burner! 2. Rinse out beakers and test tubes. 3. Return all chemicals to shelves. 4. Wipe down counter. 5. Check and write homework. 6. Turn in lab results. 7. Pack bag.	**Steps**	**Estimated time**	**Actual time**
	Step 1		
	Step 2		
	Step 3		
	Step 4		
	Step 5		
	Step 6		
	Step 7		
Did I miss any steps?	Total		

FIGURE 3.11. Worksheet for the Recipe for Success activity, extended to science lab cleanup.

Teaching Prioritizing Strategies

Teachers can help students to prioritize activities and efficiently manage time by teaching them the importance of predicting how long an activity will take and deciding how to arrange activities in their daily, weekly, or monthly schedules. By providing students with a clear understanding of the different types of activities (obligation, aspiration, and negotiation) in their daily lives, teachers can offer a method of prioritization that results in the creation of a productive and efficient schedule.

Elementary School

Setting priorities can be a difficult task for younger students, who frequently fill their schedules with activities of interest rather than independently incorporating obligatory tasks. Although it may not be developmentally appropriate to expect all elementary school students to prioritize their activities independently, it is appropriate to engage in discussions about the nature of students' daily activities. Teachers may begin by identifying the qualities that distinguish tasks (i.e., time-sensitive vs. flexible, required vs. optional), and then modeling the application of this knowledge by working with the students to create a productive daily schedule.

• *Obligation, aspiration, or negotiation?* Students can expand on their scheduler responsibilities (see earlier discussion) by helping to plan the day's schedule. Rather than having the agenda on the board when students enter the classroom, teachers can model the way in which they schedule each school day in a stepwise approach as follows:

1. Review the characteristics of each of the three forms of prioritizing: *Have to Do, Wanna do,* and *Trade?* (i.e., *obligation, aspiration,* and *negotiation*).
2. Next, place each daily class activity into one of the three groups; be sure to clearly state the reason for each decision.
3. Finally, arrange the schedule by placing obligation activities first (e.g., reading circle, math block), then scheduling aspiration activities (e.g., choice time), and lastly filling in with negotiation activities (e.g., extra recess).

Middle School

In middle school, teachers can support the development of time management skills by integrating students' burgeoning knowledge of task time estimation with an understanding of prioritization. By offering students opportunities to practice these skills in isolation before they must apply them to a larger assignment, teachers will provide a platform from which the students can sharpen their planning and prioritizing abilities without the added pressure of academic performance.

• *Obligation, aspiration, or negotiation?* In the middle school version of this activity, students can be asked to create lists of daily activities based on (1) their own schedules, (2) the imagined tasks of a historical personality (e.g., Thomas Jefferson), or (3) the responsibilities of a fictionalized character (e.g., Harry Potter). Once the list is complete, students can use the Obligation, Aspiration, and Negotiation Worksheet (Figure 3.12) to divide the tasks into categories and then to estimate the amount of time needed for each task.

• *Scheduling tasks.* In order to apply students' knowledge about prioritization to their own schedules, a calendar activity can be combined with the Obligation, Aspiration, or Negotiation Worksheet. Once activities have been assigned their appropriate level of priority and times have been estimated for each task, a calendar can provide a visual representation of how much time each of the activities will consume.

A planner (like the daily schedule shown in Figure 3.13, which is broken down by hours) can be helpful for organizing a student's day. Students can be given the following five steps to guide them through the process of planning their day:

Obligation, Aspiration, and Negotiation Worksheet			
Task	Type	Predicted Time	Actual Time
Soccer practice	Obligation	45 minutes	
Study vocabulary	Obligation	30 minutes	
Watch TV	Aspiration	30 minutes	
Math homework	Obligation	45 minutes	
Poem for Mom	Negotiation	1 hour	

FIGURE 3.12. Sample worksheet for prioritizing tasks.

1. Block off the times for waking up, school, meals, and bedtime for each day during the week.
2. Insert the obligation tasks and their allotted times from the Obligation, Aspiration, and Negotiation Worksheet (see Figure 3.12) completed earlier. It is best to use a red marker for obligation tasks, to emphasize their importance (in Figure 3.13, these tasks are given in boldface).
3. Find times for aspiration tasks.
4. Insert negotiation activities in any available slots.
5. As a last step, use the extra column to check off tasks when they have

Daily Schedule	
7:00 A.M.	BREAKFAST AND SHOWER
8:00 A.M.	**SCHOOL**
9:00 A.M.	
10:00 A.M.	
11:00 A.M.	
12:00 P.M.	
1:00 P.M.	
2:00 P.M.	
3:00 P.M.	
4:00 P.M.	**SOCCER PRACTICE**
5:00 P.M.	TV
6:00 P.M.	DINNER
7:00 P.M.	**MATH HOMEWORK**
8:00 P.M.	**STUDY VOCABULARY**
9:00 P.M.	*POEM FOR MOTHER'S DAY*
10:00 P.M.	BEDTIME

FIGURE 3.13. Sample daily schedule. Boldface indicates obligation tasks, underlining indicates aspiration tasks, and *italics* indicates negotiation tasks.

been completed. Any incomplete tasks should be moved to the next day's activities.

High School

High school students usually demonstrate a good understanding of how to categorize their tasks, but struggle to create a balanced schedule in which they allot adequate time to complete large-scale assignments. Three weeks may seem like a long time to write a paper, but when a student is faced with a calendar already filled with sports practice, vacation, and additional school responsibilities, it is easy to see how opportunities for homework are limited. Working backward is a particularly effective strategy with longer-term projects, because it provides students with a tangible representation of the steps involved and amount of time available to complete a complex assignment.

• *Working backward.* Working backward entails first placing all known obligations for a given month on the calendar (vacations, extracurricular activities, additional academic assignments, etc.). Next, students can focus on the project at hand. They should enter the due date in a way that draws attention and acts as a reminder, and then reverse the steps necessary for completion in order to identify and schedule all of the components involved with the assignment (see Figure 3.14). Most students will benefit from initially completing a Project Breakdown Work-

Monthly Calendar						
		1	2	3	4 To Kill a Mockingbird assigned	5 Soccer tournament
6 Soccer tournament	7 Read 1 hr	8 Read 2 hrs	9 Read 1 hr	10 Read 2 hrs	11 Trip to Maine	12 Trip to Maine
13 Read 1 hr	14 Write 1 hr	15 Soccer tournament	16 Write 2 hrs	17 Write 2 hrs, including editing	18 Essay on To Kill a Mocking-bird due	19
20	21	22	23	24	25	26
27	28					

FIGURE 3.14. Working backward with a monthly calendar.

sheet (see Figure 3.9) and then working backward to fill in a calendar with the previously identified steps.

Teaching Monitoring Strategies for Time Management

One of the most challenging aspects of teaching students time management skills is motivating them to change their current behaviors. One way to do this is by demonstrating to them the ways in which their current organizational choices are negatively affecting their performance. Utilizing activities that scaffold student reflection can be important tools in the behavioral process of change.

Elementary and Middle School

The final and most important step in task estimation is the revision process. Even younger students should always be aware of how well their estimated schedule aligns with the actual elapsed time, and should be supported in making any necessary revisions to ensure that they do not run out of time before completing the project. There are opportunities for elementary and middle school students to monitor their developing time managements skills in many of the activities suggested in the planning and prioritizing section of this chapter. For example, students have an opportunity to practice their monitoring skills in the Recipe for Success activity (see Figure 3.10 and 3.11), in which the activity is structured so that the individual or pair who plans the recipe, identifies each step, and estimates the time for each component is not the individual or pair who executes the recipe. (To ensure that the task is developmentally appropriate, elementary school teachers can fill in certain portions of the worksheet.) After the worksheet has been completed, it is passed to another team of students for the recipe to be carried out. In order to convey the importance of revising estimates and monitoring progress, teachers should instruct students to end the task at the estimated time, no matter where they are in the process. This exchange allows dialogue to occur between students about the accuracy of initial planning and estimates. Students can learn how to use the data they collect on their worksheets to revise their estimates.

High School

Many high school students struggle with feelings of disappointment or hopelessness over their academic performance. Often they report feeling overwhelmed and distressed as a result of unsatisfactory performance, but are unable to identify how or where to make changes. For students who are disappointed about the outcomes of large-scale assignments, worksheets that highlight where failures in planning and prioritizing occurred will provide insight into the time management skills that need to be refined.

- *Activity reflection worksheets and rubrics.* As students mature, they may no longer utilize graphic organizers. Instead, older students may benefit from special journals in which they can keep organized records of completed tasks, document their satisfaction with the outcomes, and comment about possible areas for future improvement. Ideally, when they maintain these structured records and reflections, the students' own feedback will be organized in a way that will reveal patterns of behavior and aid them in improving their time management skills over the school year. The worksheets provided in Figures 3.15 and 3.16 constitute a semistructured activity that helps students to analyze how organizational and time management strategies can affect both their academic and nonacademic performance.

CONCLUSION

Today, probably more than ever, educators are being asked to respond to rapid changes in the social, economic, and technological arenas by preparing children to solve new problems in our world. As they juggle their many responsibilities and challenges, it is critically important for teachers to systematically teach students strategies for setting goals, planning, and prioritizing. Teachers facing these tasks can take heart: They already know what it takes to be effective in the classroom, since they understand the importance of direct, systematic, explicit instruction. They only need to extend this understanding beyond the traditional areas of reading, spelling, and math. In addition, it is important for teachers to recognize that

Activity Reflection Worksheet				
Type of assignment and date	Did you prioritize your taks?	Did you accurately estimate how long each task would take?	Did you revise your schedule when it was necessary?	Did you delegate or delete less important tasks to accomplish the activities that were most important?
History test 10/13/10	Yes	No	Yes	Yes
CHANGES FOR NEXT TIME				
Please describe why your schedule did not work.		Underestimated the amount of time it would take. I estimated 1 hour and it was not long enough.		
Please describe how your schedule can be improved in the future.		Next time I study, I will for 2 hours over 2 days (1 hour per day).		

FIGURE 3.15. Sample activity reflection sheet.

Reflection Rubric			
Name of assigment/task:		Outcome: (Example: grade, performance, etc.)	
How well was your time managed?			
1 Not Well	2 Sort of Well	3 Well	4 Very Well
____ Did not prioritize ____ Did not estimate accurately ____ Procrastinated ____ Ultimately had to sacrifice many things I wanted to do, because I was overwhelmed by my schedule	____ Prioritized ____ Did no estimate accuately ____ Ran out of time ____ Could have done with more time	____ Prioritized ____ Estimated accuately ____ Mostly followed plan ____ Did not revise, delegate, or delete activities when unexpected opportunities arose ____ In the end, still felt stressed and frustrated	____ Prioritized ____ Estimated accurately ____ Followed through with plan ____ Revised schedule when necessary ____ Delegated/deleted less imp. activites and felt satisfied with use of time
Which area of time management should I concentrate on next time? ____ Prioritizing ____ Estimating ____ Revising ____ Delegating/deleting *Comments:* Which areas of time management does my teacher think I should concentrate on next time? ____ Prioritizing ____ Estimating ____ Revising ____ Delegating/deleting *Comments:*			

FIGURE 3.16. Sample reflection rubric.

they can be highly successful in teaching strategies for goal setting, planning, and prioritizing when they:

- Embed strategies for goal setting, planning, and prioritizing within the curriculum.
- Allocate sufficient time for students to learn and practice their strategies.
- Teach the *what, why,* and *how* of using strategies for goal setting, planning, and prioritizing.

CHAPTER 4

Organizing

The Heart of Efficient and Successful Learning

KALYANI KRISHNAN and MELISSA J. FELLER

Science is organized knowledge. Wisdom is organized life.
—IMMANUEL KANT

Lisa walks into her room, which looks as if it has experienced a tornado. She looks around for a minute trying to find a clean pair of socks, abandons her search, and leaves for school in a pair of flip-flops. At school, she opens her locker, and several books fall out. She is late for class because of the time it takes her to repack her locker. She smiles apologetically at her annoyed teacher and takes her seat.

Bob's mind is a whirl of ideas. There is so much to share with his mom. When he sees her, the words spill out of his mouth, but his mother only looks at him in confusion and asks, "What on earth are you trying to tell me about?" This is not a new experience. Bob has always struggled to convey his ideas to others, and his attempts often end in frustrated silence or tears.

Lisa and Bob embody some of the traits and behaviors that we recognize as constituting "poor organization." According to common dictionary definitions, *organization* is ordering parts into a cohesive whole so that they can collectively serve a common goal. Lisa struggles to order her materials so that she can find what she needs in an efficient manner. Bob, on the other hand, struggles to order his thoughts and ideas into a cohesive narrative so that he can communicate his ideas effectively.

In this chapter, we discuss the executive function processes involved in organization, and describe strategies for promoting the development of these important processes at the elementary, middle, and high school levels. Specifically, we focus on strategies for supporting students' ability to organize their learning environments and materials. We also discuss strategies for helping students to organize expository and narrative information. The strategies and techniques described in this chapter have been drawn from a variety of sources. Where they are based on scientific evidence, we provide the appropriate references, including empirical and clinical studies. Many strategies we describe have been highly effective in clinical practice but have not yet been evaluated in experimental studies; nonetheless, they are offered as ideas for the reader's consideration and for future directions in educational research.

WHY IS IT IMPORTANT TO TEACH ORGANIZATIONAL STRATEGIES SYSTEMATICALLY?

The executive function processes involved in organization are mediated by the frontal lobes and are subject to developmental trends (Huttenlocher & Dabholkar, 1997; Thatcher, 1997). As with other biologically based processes (e.g., language development), we can assume that they are also distributed normally in the population. In any age group, there is considerable variation in students' abilities to organize materials and ideas. Some students acquire the necessary organizational skills to become successful, independent learners quickly and easily, while others need explicit teaching and more opportunities for practice. An analogy is provided by examining the field of reading. Although many children appear to acquire reading skills simply through exposure to print and engagement with the activity of reading, research has shown that reading is a complex process that can be easily disrupted by processing difficulties in any number of areas, including attention, memory, and language (Shaywitz, 2003). Thus, whereas some children learn to read easily, many others need a highly explicit, systematic curriculum (Adams, 1999; Shaywitz, 2003). At the same time, *all* children benefit from exposure to the rules of phonics in a developmentally sequenced manner. Similarly, at school meetings we have attended, many teachers have voiced the assumption that children will learn organizational skills when they are placed in an organized environment or have these skills and strategies modeled for them. However, our clinical experience suggests that organization is also a multifaceted and complex process, and that all students may benefit from systematic instruction and strategies. Furthermore, many children *need* explicit, systematic, and structured strategy instruction to organize their environment, materials, and ideas.

Moreover, recent changes in public education have raised expectations for independence, analysis, and synthesis of information, as well as written productivity, in children as young as kindergartners. All of these skills require the fluent and efficient deployment of executive function processes, particularly organizational strategies. The recent reliance on high-stakes testing has fueled this movement.

As a result, young children in grades 1–3, who may not be developmentally ready to meet the layered demands of long-term projects, are being asked to complete month-long book reports and projects with minimal teacher support. However, students are not being taught systematically to organize information so that they can identify the different parts of the project, and then integrate the parts back into a cohesive whole once each element is completed. In other words, if we are asking young children to complete tasks that rely on executive function processes such as organization, we need to teach these strategies explicitly and systematically in the early grades.

Explicit instruction in organizational strategies is particularly necessary for students with learning and/or attention difficulties, who often experience difficulties with the executive function processes involved in organizing their school materials and the information they are learning (Kops & Belmont, 1985; Meltzer & Krishnan, 2007). Our clinical experience indicates that school personnel do recognize the need for directly teaching organizational skills in the middle grades. Many middle schools offer study skills courses and have specific expectations that students maintain organized binders and fill out agenda books. Thus students are expected to learn the skills and strategies they need at the same time as they are expected to apply them. Experienced teachers and clinicians know that students with vulnerabilities in the processes that underlie independent learning (i.e., attention, memory, language, and executive function) need sufficient time to learn, practice, integrate, and generalize these skills before they are required to function independently. Therefore, teaching organizational strategies systematically in the early grades is important for all students and is crucial for those with learning and/or attention difficulties (Meltzer, 1993; Swanson, 1989). When organizational strategies are explicitly and sequentially taught from the early grades on, teachers will be more likely to "catch" students with vulnerabilities. Furthermore, those students who need more time to practice the necessary strategies and build their organizational skills incrementally will be afforded this opportunity.

Finally, our clinical experience shows that when students are expected to meet the organizational demands of their learning environment before they are sufficiently equipped, they may experience feelings of frustration, anxiety, and overload, making it even more challenging for them to keep pace with academic demands. In addition, feelings of anxiety and fatigue can impair higher-level cortical functions, which include the executive function processes needed for organizing thinking and solving problems (Caine & Caine, 2006). Therefore, explicitly teaching organizational strategies across the grades will help students acquire a strong repertoire of strategies that will enhance their ability to:

- Successfully access the materials they need to complete their work.
- Store information they are learning.
- Express the ideas and concepts they have learned.

- Select organizational strategies that are appropriate for the task or situation.
- Understand their learning profiles and choose the organizational strategies that work for them.

WHAT FOUNDATIONAL SKILLS ARE INVOLVED IN ACQUIRING ORGANIZATIONAL STRATEGIES?

In order to organize school materials, information, and ideas for greater independence in the academic setting, students need to acquire the ability to:

- Understand the current structure of the learning environment and interpret task expectations.
- Sort and classify information from the concrete to the conceptual level.
- Select and utilize appropriate organizational strategies.
- Reflect on the effectiveness of these strategies.

Understanding the Existing Environmental Structure and Task Expectations

To become successful organizers in school, students must first recognize how their learning environment is structured. *Schema theory* suggests that individuals process complex situations by using their previously encoded general knowledge about similar situations (Matlin, 2002). A schema is a framework of information that is created when something new is learned (Sweller, van Merrienboer, & Paas, 1998). It consists of a gestalt of the knowledge or experience including a network of connected facts and perceptions, as well as internalized scripts. Each new related experience expands and further integrates the original schema. This network of knowledge is stored in long-term memory and provides a way for new experiences and information to be interpreted within the context of known schemas. For example, students who have been on one field trip know what to expect on the second one (e.g., a permission slip needs to be signed, a bag lunch is needed, there may be a long bus ride, the teachers may sing songs with them on the bus). Thus, as students are afforded explicit opportunities to develop strong schemas for the organization of their learning, they will be able to allocate the needed cognitive resources efficiently as they engage in the lessons being taught.

Sorting and Classifying Information

In addition to understanding the structure of the learning environment and the task at hand, it is crucial for students to be able to sort and classify concrete, conceptual, and abstract information. Just as students may have preferences for one sensory modality over another (e.g., visual learners, auditory learners, tactile learners), they may also show either a "top-down" style or a "bottom-up" approach. Top-down processors tend to see the "big picture" first. For example, they may organize information they have brainstormed for a writing assignment by creating major categories and then filling in details relevant to those categories. Bottom-up processors tend to start with the details and then shift to the major categories. With either approach, students need to move flexibly between the big picture and relevant details as new information becomes available. Lastly, students need to employ these strategies for categorizing at both a concrete level (e.g., sorting and organizing tangible materials, such as papers in a binder) and a conceptual level (e.g., planning a persuasive essay).

Selecting from a Repertoire of Organizational Strategies

In a review of over two decades of research, Gettinger and Seibert (2002) found that success in academic content areas is often directly linked to effective study strategies. In the organizational realm, students must have a variety of strategies at their disposal, and know where, when, and how to use them (Meltzer et al., 2006). In other words, students must develop a repertoire of organizational strategies (see Chapters 1 and 2). By learning and practicing several such strategies, students begin to understand what works best in relation to their unique learning styles and their individual strengths and weaknesses. Given the multiple demands that students must manage on a daily basis, there is no "one size fits all" organizational strategy for all tasks and learning situations. Moreover, the diverse learners in today's classrooms come to school with a wide variety of intellectual and physical skills. Therefore, all students need the opportunity to learn and practice strategies that will promote their ability to manage their own learning.

Engaging in Self-Reflection

Lastly, to use strategies independently, students need to reflect on the effectiveness of the strategies that they have chosen. In doing so, they need to learn how to select the appropriate strategy or strategies for each specific task's demands from their repertoire, and how to adjust these strategies to make them more useful in the future. A painter uses different brushes to obtain desired effects on the canvas, and a chef does not use the same ingredients for every recipe. Similarly, students need to select appropriate organizational strategies on the basis of prior knowledge, or *hindsight*, as well as an understanding of the task at hand and the possible outcomes, or *forethought* ("What is likely to happen?"), in order to become independent organizers (Ward, 2007). By planning their approaches in these ways, students can choose organizational strategies that best fit their learning styles. A sample Strategy Reflection Sheet is provided in Appendix 4.

HOW SHOULD ORGANIZATIONAL STRATEGIES BE TAUGHT?

Tell me and I'll forget; show me and I may remember;
involve me and I'll understand.
—CHINESE PROVERB

The basic principles for strategy instruction are detailed in Chapter 2. In addition to these principles, effective strategy instruction for organizing needs to be systematically implemented starting in the early grades, with foundational strategies laying the groundwork for more layered and nuanced strategies in the later grades. As children mature, control over strategy selection and application can be gradually relinquished through a scaffolded process, so that students are better equipped to handle the increased responsibility for more independent learning at the upper grades and into adulthood. Table 4.1 provides a proposed developmental progression for teaching organizational strategies that facilitates students' integration, generalization, and independent deployment of these strategies. It is important to note that not all students will need the same level of support through the grades, as some students will become self-regulated and metacognitive earlier than others. Therefore, teachers need to differentiate their instruction to address the individual needs of their students. The developmental progression provides a framework for understanding how individual students fit into the continuum of learning organizational strategies.

As Table 4.1 suggests, it is very important that structured, systematic, school-wide approaches be created and used to promote the development of organizational strategies across the grades (see Chapters 1 and 2). By weaving explicit instruction in organizational strategies into the everyday curriculum consistently from grade to grade, teachers can build students' ability to develop organizational schemas for materials and ideas.

TABLE 4.1. Developmental Progression for Teaching Organizational Strategies

Age level	Concept	Methodology
Elementary school	Model strategies	• Provide explicit instruction and guided practice. • Provide systematic spiraling and review of strategies. • Have students develop strategy notebooks.
Middle school	Promote independence	• Continue guided practice and cueing to promote independence. • Systematic spiraling and review. • Have students maintain and add to strategy notebooks.
High school	Support independence	• Continue cueing until strategies are fully integrated and internalized. • Encourage students to personalize strategies. • Continue to encourage use of strategy notebooks as needed.

To begin shaping organizational strategies in the classroom, it is important to apply the following broad principles:

• *Use consistent routines to ensure predictability.* When classroom routines are predictable, and students become self-sufficient in navigating these routines, they can allocate more cognitive resources to learning the content. Routines can be established for entering and exiting the classroom, managing supplies, engaging in cooperative or individual work, recording and turning in homework assignments, and structuring instructional time. For example, to establish a routine for recording homework, a teacher can designate a location on a blackboard or bulletin board as the place where homework assignments are posted. At a designated time, students are taught to take out their assignment notebooks, look at the "homework spot," and record the day's assignments. If there is no homework, students write "none" in their notebooks.

• *Provide sufficient time for organization.* Teachers should take time at the beginning of the year to establish routines, create goals for organizing, and model targeted organizational behaviors. Doing so will decrease the frequent interruptions caused by hunts for lost or misplaced materials, searches for missing homework, and the need to redirect students who are "off track." As students become more proficient with the routines established in the classroom, they will be more efficient and will be able to spend more time on task.

• *Apply thoughtful cueing.* Cueing that guides students to approach tasks systematically and strategically is important for fostering greater independence with tasks requiring organization and problem solving. For example, for long-range projects, teachers can cue students with the types of questions that should be helpful as students plan their approach. The following examples are based on the work of Marlowe (2000). The language used may need to be modified to meet the developmental levels of individual students.

> "What are you trying to accomplish?"
> "What steps are involved?"
> "What might be possible barriers to accomplishing this task?"
> "What strategies can you use in order to complete this assignment?"
> "What materials are you going to need?"
> "How will you know when you are completely finished?"
> "What can you do to make sure that you have met all of the expectations?"

• *Compile strategies.* Using strategy notebooks to compile organizational strategies for later use helps students to recognize how their repertoire is growing and provides them with concrete resources that can be used during learning activities. Chapter 2 has described the use of personal strategy notebooks. Students can compile the organizational strategies that work best for them in these notebooks. Teachers can cue students to refer to their notebooks when opportunities arise, which will help build the important metacognitive skills necessary for employing organizational strategies effectively. The strategy notebooks will also help students to track their strategies to see how their repertoire has grown.

WHAT SPECIFIC ORGANIZATIONAL STRATEGIES SHOULD BE TAUGHT EXPLICITLY?

Teachers can foster the foundational skills discussed in preceding sections by teaching students organizational strategies in two broad areas:

1. Organizing space and materials.
2. Organizing ideas (expository and narrative information).

Organizing Space and Materials

In this section, we address ways in which teachers can guide students to access existing supports and structures in their environment, so that they can go on to develop more personalized organizational strategies.

Elementary School

In the early grades (grades K–3), the majority of teachers present their students with highly structured environments. Any visitor to a typical early elementary classroom will recall the bright colors and clearly marked stations. In addition, discussions about the calendar, schedule, and daily activities are built into the daily routine and typically take place "on the rug," or during classroom meetings early in the day. It is therefore surprising when students emerge from these early grades with highly variable skills in organizing their own space and materials. Observations and discussions with elementary-grade teachers suggest that the teachers are the ones who take the lead and responsibility for creating the structure, and that students are only consumers of the existing structure. Thus, although students are given an explicit structure, they may not internalize it. The following steps are recommended to facilitate young students' internalization and generalization of organizational structures.

• *Describe the structure.* During the first several weeks of school, the teacher and students can discuss the organization of the classroom space and materials. Students can "interview" the teacher to understand why he or she has set things up in that particular way, and then explain what they have learned to their classmates.

• *Use the structure consistently.* Students can practice using the existing structure, and teachers can promote independence, by strategically prompting students to think about broad categories. For example, if a student loses pencils or paper, the teacher can use this opportunity to cue for independent problem solving. (STUDENT: "I don't have a pencil." TEACHER: "Where do we store tools in our classroom?") Similarly, if students need help with spelling specific words, the teacher can prompt them to find a dictionary by looking among the reference materials.

• *Evaluate the structure.* As students become familiar with the existing structure, the teacher can periodically initiate discussions that encourage students to evaluate the structure within the class. These discussions can take place as whole-class conversations, in small groups, or with individual students. Some guiding questions might include these:

> "Does it work?"
> "Why does it work?"
> "Are there any problems?"

• *Adjust the structure.* On the basis of the class consensus or feedback, the students can collectively devise solutions for their problems.

• *Create anew.* During the second half of the year, the teacher can require the class to revamp the structure of the classroom as a collective project. If this is too big a project, a single aspect of organization may be selected for students to think about, plan, and implement (e.g., setting up the reading corner in a new way that makes sense). For example, some elementary teachers have students organize the classroom libraries by categorizing books into labeled bins.

As students progress into the upper elementary grades, teachers can build upon what students have learned about organizing their space with the following steps:

• Initiate a classwide discussion about organization and how it works (this taps metacognition).

> "What do you know about organizing?"
> "Why is organizing important?"
> "Are there different ways to organize?"

• Initiate a class discussion about styles of learning and help students to understand their preferred organizational style (this taps self-knowledge).

• Have students organize their desks and materials in a way that matches their needs (e.g., one student may color-code, another may need additional space). Alternatively, students can work in pairs to solve problems collaboratively.

Following this, students need to apply the first four critical metacognitive steps described above to fine-tune their organization:

- *Say how to organize* (i.e., describe the structure). For example, a student might say, "OK, I'm organizing my desk. First I need to make groups of things that go together. I can put the papers in my folder. Extra pencils can go in my pencil case. My crayons need to go in the box . . . "
  - *Use the structure consistently.*
  - *Evaluate the structure*: "Is it working or not?"
  - *Adjust the structure*: "How can I make it work better?"

One way of remembering this structure is for students and teachers to use the first letter of each step above to create an acronym that helps the children remember the steps for organizing. Say, Use, Evaluate, and Adjust yields the acronym SUE-A.

Say, Use, Evaluate, and Adjust: SUE-A
Who helps us organize? SUE-A helps us organize!

Middle School

As we have suggested earlier in this chapter (see especially Table 4.1), students in middle school still need guided practice and cueing to a great extent. Many students enter middle school with some awareness of their preferred organizational styles, while many others experience significant difficulties with the increased demands for independence at this level. One challenge for many students is the way they manage their lockers. Incoming middle school students may benefit from models and explicit examples of the ways in which they can organize their lockers. Once different ways of organizing lockers have been shown to students, they can choose a method and try it. Again, students can use SUE-A: They can *verbalize* their method (*say* it aloud), *use* it consistently, *evaluate* its effectiveness over time, and *adjust* the system to match their individual learning styles.

High School

Although students in high school typically make independent choices about ways of organizing their materials and space, teachers can continue to reinforce the critical metacognitive steps in the upper grades. For students who continue to need explicit support, teachers can use the methods suggested for middle school. These students may need extra time to practice the strategies before teacher support is completely relinquished.

Using the metacognitive steps described above, teachers can help their students approach a range of other organizational challenges relative to organizing space and materials. A set of sample strategies that teachers can use to help students strategically approach the management of papers is provided in Table 4.2.

TABLE 4.2. Sample Strategies for Managing Papers: A Developmental Progression

Grade level	Strategies and systems
Elementary school	• Teach students to date every paper given. • Teach students to maintain a folder for bringing papers to and from school. • Check weekly to make sure backpacks and folders are in order. • Give feedback weekly on whether student is meeting expectations and on track.
Middle school	• Continue to require students to date every paper they are given. • Model two or three effective systems for organizing papers. Require students to choose and use one system consistently. • Use composition notebooks instead of loose-leaf paper for class notes, to minimize lost papers. • Apply SUE-A (see text). • Check weekly to make sure backpacks and folders are in order. • Give feedback weekly on whether students are meeting expectations. • Hold students accountable for keeping their systems in order.
High school	• Continue to cue students to date every paper, every day. • For students who struggle, continue middle-school-level support until they are independent.

Again, teachers need to consider students' individual needs when determining which strategies and systems the students should be expected to apply and with what level of support.

Organizing Ideas

Students' ability to organize information and to express ideas in order to "show what they know" hinges on an important foundational skill: *sorting and categorizing concepts*. Teachers can facilitate categorization across grade levels by providing opportunities for students to learn strategies for sorting, beginning at a concrete level and moving gradually to a more conceptual level.

In preschool and early elementary school, children often participate in activities that require them to sort concrete objects and familiar ideas (e.g., animals, rocks, the weather, etc.). During such activities, students will benefit from practicing both bottom-up and top-down strategies for sorting (regardless of their natural preference), as this promotes flexibility. A worksheet for sorting activities is provided in Appendix 5 (see Figure 4.1 for a completed example).

Often, despite engaging in varied sorting activities, many students have difficulty categorizing information at a conceptual level—a process that is critical for successful reading comprehension, as well as oral and written expression. However, with explicit strategy instruction, teachers can begin to lay the foundation for the organization of ideas from the earliest grades by teaching students to appreciate how spoken and written discourses are structured. A fundamental distinction in the way information is organized is seen when comparing narrative and expository formats. The common traits of each of these formats are illustrated in Figure 4.2. Teachers are encouraged to initiate discussions about these organizing

Work with your team members to sort your group of items, pictures, or words into three to six categories. Write your answers in the boxes below. Then fill out your reflection.

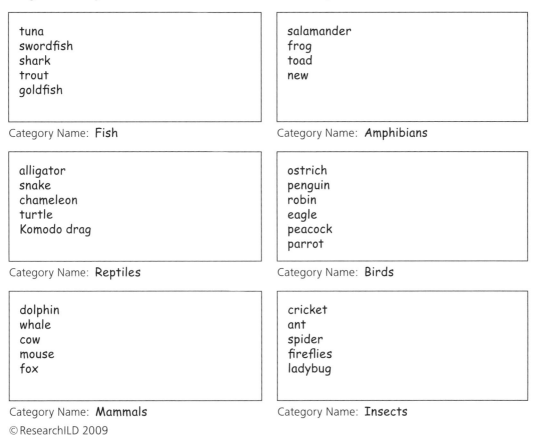

tuna swordfish shark trout goldfish	salamander frog toad new
Category Name: **Fish**	Category Name: **Amphibians**
alligator snake chameleon turtle Komodo drag	ostrich penguin robin eagle peacock parrot
Category Name: **Reptiles**	Category Name: **Birds**
dolphin whale cow mouse fox	cricket ant spider fireflies ladybug
Category Name: **Mammals**	Category Name: **Insects**

© ResearchILD 2009

FIGURE 4.1. A completed example of a worksheet for sorting activities (see Appendix 5).

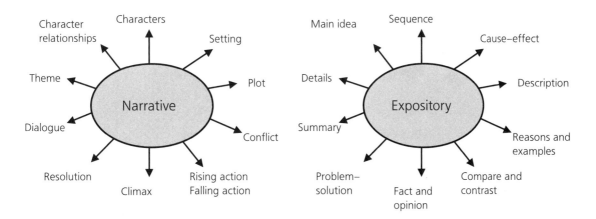

Narrative: Character relationships, Characters, Setting, Theme, Plot, Dialogue, Conflict, Resolution, Climax, Rising action / Falling action

Expository: Main idea, Sequence, Cause–effect, Details, Description, Summary, Reasons and examples, Problem–solution, Fact and opinion, Compare and contrast

FIGURE 4.2. Teaching organizational strategies for narrative versus expository discourse.

features as early as possible, using some of the strategies that we describe in the next few pages.

Expository Information

EARLY ELEMENTARY SCHOOL (GRADES K–3)

In the early grades, teachers can foster students' ability to *distinguish between main ideas and details*—a key foundational skill for comprehending and composing expository text. One way teachers in the elementary grades can facilitate this is by using pictures to help students infer main ideas (bottom-up tasks). In the same way, teachers can use pictures to help students generate detail statements (top-down tasks). Sample activities are described below:

Bottom-Up Tasks

One way pictures can be used to teach younger children to extract main ideas is to present an array of related pictures along with several possible main-idea statements (see Figures 4.3 and 4.4). Students engage in discussions to determine what all of the pictures have in common (i.e., analyze the details). The students then consider the statements provided and select the one that best expresses the main idea. The level of scaffolding can be altered, depending upon students' needs. For example, once students become adept at recognizing the main-idea statement from a multiple-choice array, they can generate their own main-idea statements after comparing sets of pictures.

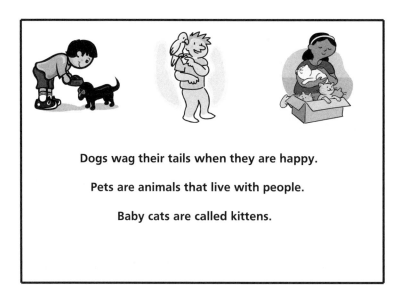

Dogs wag their tails when they are happy.

Pets are animals that live with people.

Baby cats are called kittens.

FIGURE 4.3. Bottom-up task for differentiating main ideas. Created by Paula DiPerri, Richer Elementary School. Reprinted with permission.

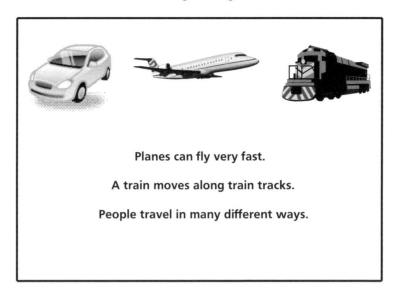

Planes can fly very fast.

A train moves along train tracks.

People travel in many different ways.

FIGURE 4.4. Bottom-up task for differentiating main ideas. Created by Paula DiPerri, Richer Elementary School.

Top-Down Tasks

Teachers can choose pictures, such as the one by Norman Rockwell described in Figure 4.5, to facilitate a top-down approach to generating details. Using such a picture as an anchor, a teacher can give the picture a title (main idea) and then elicit details and inferences from students through guided questions. The discussion will allow the class to judge the appropriateness of details and inferences. As the students become proficient in generating relevant details and drawing accurate inferences, the teacher can fade away the guiding questions and ask students to generate their own questions. Once all the questions have been answered, the students can discuss why the title was appropriate, given the details they generated.

The following are sample questions to use with Norman Rockwell's "Four Sporting Boys—Oh Yeah," a vibrant scene depicting boys who have momentarily paused their basketball game to dispute their opponents' point of view.

- Who are these children?
- Where are they?
- What are they doing?
- How do you feel?
- What happened just before?
- What might happen next?

FIGURE 4.5. Top-down task for differentiating main ideas.

The STAR strategy mentioned in Chapter 2 provides a scaffold for helping students develop a range of question types. This task is an important precursor to more advanced reading comprehension and writing tasks. Scaffolding can also be faded by having students generate their own titles as a whole-class activity, and students can then vote for the one they like best. Once again, teachers can help students to think critically by making a case for their favorite title.

Last, elementary students can begin to organize information by learning common patterns present in expository discourse, such as those:

- Describing an event or item.
- Explaining how to do something.
- Listing information in a sequence (e.g., "first . . . , second . . . , third . . . , finally . . . ").
- Discussing causes and effects.
- Discussing reasons or examples to support a statement (e.g., "Our school is great for many reasons").
- Determining similarities and differences between two things (e.g., "There are similarities between alligators and crocodiles").

Teachers can begin by selecting texts that follow these patterns and providing students with opportunities to recognize clues that help distinguish one pattern from another. Once students become skilled at recognizing these patterns in reading material relevant to the content they are learning, they can begin to apply the patterns to their own writing. There are many templates available to help students organize information according to these common patterns (see, e.g., Jennings & Haynes, 2002). When they learn how language is commonly structured for spoken and written communication, students will more easily make the transition to the formal writing requirements of middle and high school.

UPPER ELEMENTARY, MIDDLE, AND HIGH SCHOOL (GRADES 4 AND UP)

To promote the ability to sort, categorize, and organize at the conceptual level in the upper grades, teachers can provide students with various opportunities to categorize information that has been taught. Doing this can help tie together themes that have been introduced, as well as promote an appreciation of the connections between content areas, across time periods, and so on. Here are some examples:

"What do all of the novels we have read this year have in common?"
"In what ways was the system of government in the Roman Empire similar to our government today?"
"How do scientists use categories when describing the planets of our solar system?"

Sorting for Meaning: Vocabulary

Semantic feature charts can be introduced to help students understand relationships between concepts they are learning by looking at similarities and differences according to particular comparison–contrast criteria (see Figure 4.6). Semantic mapping strategies are also helpful for enriching students' study of vocabulary beyond simply memorizing definitions and using new words in novel sentences. Students can pair up and brainstorm, categorize, label the categories, and discuss the words and concepts related to a target word. This promotes connections between and among content areas and fosters development of theme recognition, which is critical for advanced reading comprehension. In fact, research has shown that students

Types of rock	Formed by magma	Formed by heat and pressure	Formed by other rocks
Granite	+	–	–
Slate	–	+	–
Coal	–	–	+
Obsidian	+	–	–
Limestone	–	–	+
Shale	–	–	+
Schist	–	+	–
Gneiss	–	+	–
Sandstone	–	–	+
Gypsum	–	–	+
Pumice	+	–	–

Quadrilaterals	All sides equal	Opposite sides are parallel	Only one pair of parallel sides	All angles equal	Opposite angles equal
Parallelogram	+/–	+	–	+/–	+
Rectangle	+/–	+	–	+	+
Square	+	+	–	+	+
Rhombus	+	+	–	–	+
Trapezoid	–	–	+	–	–

Types of fiction	Animals are the main characters	People or gods are the main characters	Teaches a lesson	Provides an explanation for something in nature	Is based on some actual events
Myths	–	+	–	+	–
Legends	–	+	+/–	–	+
Folk tales	–	+	+	+/–	+
Fables	+	–	+	+_	–
Fairy tales	+/–	+/–	+/–	–	–

FIGURE 4.6. Sample semantic feature analysis grids for three different content areas.

demonstrate stronger comprehension and vocabulary learning after engaging in vocabulary instruction that includes interactive strategies, rather than instruction that solely uses definitions (Bos & Anderson, 1990). Teachers can enhance students' ability to identify and formulate main ideas and details by explicitly pointing out how the category names are the main ideas and the group items are the details.

Sorting for Meaning: Text

Students in middle and high school are often required to read, understand, and analyze expository text, as well as to express their knowledge of what they have learned in a variety of writing assignments. Teachers can continue to provide opportunities for students to practice identifying and applying organizational patterns found within expository text for both reading comprehension and written expression, while gradually reducing scaffolds. Cueing can foster self-directed organization of ideas and promote greater independence. Here are some examples:

- *For reading*:
  "What do you notice about the way the information is organized?"
  "What clues do we see?"
  "Why did the author organize the information this way?"
- *For written language*:
  "What question are you being asked to answer?"
  "How can you organize your ideas to help the reader understand your answer?"
  "Are you being asked to express your opinion, compare two things, or give an explanation?"

Organizing for Reading Comprehension and Writing

Identifying the Main Idea. Structured and frequent practice with identifying main ideas within paragraphs is an excellent warm-up activity for the classroom. Using texts from a variety of sources for this activity helps students become familiar with the format of different types of sources (e.g., textbooks vs. articles). They also become familiar with the way information is organized (e.g., the main idea is usually at the beginning of the paragraph, followed by examples; subheadings name subcategories of the main topic of the chapter). This enables students to use their printed resources more effectively when reading (e.g., "If I don't understand the main idea, I should look later in the paragraph for examples").

When main ideas are not explicitly stated, teachers can guide students to look for common themes, just as they have done during sorting and classifying activities. Again, modeling and cueing that target the thinking *process* will be most effective for helping students to generalize these skills to independent learning situations. Students should be prompted to consider whether the main idea they have chosen is too specific, too general, or a "perfect fit" with the details. These and additional cueing questions are listed in Figure 4.7. For a greater degree of support, a list of possible main ideas can be provided.

Structured, multisensory, and systematic programs such as Project Read offer formalized methods for teaching strategies for language integration (Enfield & Greene, 1989). Specifically, the Project Read Report Form is an example of a field-tested method that explicitly teaches students concrete strategies for gathering information about what they are reading. It includes explicit processes for identifying the central idea, key facts, and supporting details, as well as for categorizing information to show the relationship between the central idea and smaller details. Another effective approach that helps students sort and organize ideas through active reading is *reciprocal teaching*, a scaffolded discussion technique for reading comprehension that has been shown by research to be an effective method for teaching students active reading strategies (Palincsar & Brown, 1984). This approach consists of a set of four core that students learn to help them develop their comprehension-monitoring abilities. In pairs or small groups, participants take turns assuming the roles of teacher and student while reading from a common text. After explicit instruction from a teacher, students engage in *questioning* to ensure understanding, *summarizing* to integrate information, *clarifying* additional specific questions (e.g., about vocabulary) and *predicting* to provide metacognitive scaffolds for anticipated information.

Organizing Content for Writing. Once students have mastered the essential foundational skills of sorting and classifying, they will be better equipped to differentiate and shift flexibly between main ideas and details. They will then be ready to learn explicit strategies for organizing the content of their writing. To date, scientific research has validated several specific strategies for a variety of writing genres that aid students in producing more effective writing:

Metacognitive Cueing for Determining Main Ideas

- Do you notice any words or phrases that are repeated again and again?
- How do all of the sentences relate? How are they similar, or what do they have in common?
- If you had to give a category name for these details, how would you label them?
- Does your main idea tell about all of the details, or only some of them?
- Could you make your main idea more specific?
- How did you select the main idea?

FIGURE 4.7. Metacognitive cueing for determining main ideas.

- The PLEASE strategy (Pick a topic, List your ideas about the topic, Evaluate your list, Activate the paragraph with a with a topic sentence, Supply supporting sentences, and Evaluate your list) (Welch, 1992).

- Summary writing, when explicitly taught, helps students identify important information (Nelson, Smith, & Dodd, 1992).

- A technique for brainstorming ideas before composing persuasive essays is the three-step strategy with TREE: (1) Identify audience and purpose for writing; (2) develop a plan and use TREE: Topic sentence, Reasons, Examine each reason, Ending; (3) write and continue the processing of planning while writing (Graham & Harris, 1989).

- A strategy for brainstorming the components of a persuasive essay, in order to ensure that students have presented both sides of an issue, Is STOP and DARE. STOP means Suspend judgment, Take a side, Organize ideas, and Plan more as you write. When students plan as they write, DARE provides a reminder of the four essential parts of the persuasive essay: Develop a topic sentence, Add supporting details, Reject arguments for the other side, and End with a conclusion (De La Paz & Graham, 1997).

- For writing explanatory essays or those involving comparing–contrasting, the POWER strategy (Plan, Organize, Write, Edit, Revise) provides a framework for brainstorming and organizing (Englert, Raphael, & Anderson, 1992).

The strategies listed above are well documented in the literature (Graham & Harris, 2005; Harris, Graham, Mason, & Friedlander, 2008). Furthermore, while all students benefit from exposure to a wide range of strategies, these research-based strategies will be particularly helpful to students with language, learning, and attention difficulties.

Organizing for Studying

Strong organizational strategies are critical for note taking and studying. Students often struggle to determine what information is most essential. In addition to improving students' sorting and categorizing strategies and their understanding of expository patterns, teachers can explicitly teach strategies for tackling note taking and studying. Teachers can facilitate the use of these organizational strategies by embedding them into the routines of the classroom and making them count as part of the course grade (see Chapters 1 and 2 for additional discussion).

Learning to Take Notes. Skim, RAP, Map (Meltzer et al., 2006) is an effective strategy for helping students read analytically and take notes in an organized manner (see Figure 4.8). Students first learn to *skim* the text (e.g., a history or science text), noting elements that stand out. For example, they glance over titles, headings/ subheadings, illustrations, the first and last sentence in each paragraph, summary

Skim: Look at . . .
- Chapter objectives
- Headings/subheadings
- Bold/italicized words
- Margin notes and sidebars
- All visuals and captions
- Summary questions at end of chapter

RAP
- Read all parts of each section.
- Ask questions (turn each heading and subheading into a question).
- Paraphrase.

MAP
- Set up two-column notes.
- Write the RAP questions on the left, and map the answers on the right.

FIGURE 4.8. The Skim, RAP, and map strategy.

questions at the end of each chapter, and so on. Next, students *RAP* (Read, Ask questions, Paraphrase). They turn headings into questions and locate answers as they read. Lastly, they *map* the information by writing it down in the form of two-column notes (see Figure 4.9). It is important to note that students can also record the information on index cards (using both sides of each card instead of two columns) or in a linear outline. As discussed in Chapter 2, two-column notes can be extended into a Triple Note Tote to include a column for strategies (see Figure 4.10).

Learning to Write a Thesis Statement. Many students struggle to synthesize their ideas and reach beyond the text to formulate thesis statements. The PROVE strategy (Present your knowledge, Reveal information, Offer examples or explanations, Verify your knowledge, Express your knowledge in a summary statement; Scanlon, 2002) gives students a scaffold that helps them identify concepts, provide evidence in support of their positions, consider counterarguments, and integrate their arguments into a strong thesis. See Figure 4.11 for a sample from a student. Teachers can introduce the concept of a counterargument as early as third or fourth grade in a classroom where open discussion is the norm. Thus they can lay the foundation for developing strong thesis statements and consideration of counterarguments before these skills are explicitly required by the curriculum.

Supporting the Thesis Effectively. A second strategy for expository writing that provides students with a structure and process for developing five-paragraph essays is the Pieces of a Thesis strategy (described in Meltzer et al., 2006). This

Questions	Answers
Who was Napoleon Bonaparte?	• 1800 French general whose political ambition and military skill caused fear across Europe. • Conquered neighboring countries and also dreamed of rebuilding French empire in North America, but was stopped by Toussaint's troops.
Who was Toussaint L'ouverture?	• Ruled island of Haiti which Napoleon tried to take (1802) and use as a supply base but Toussaint's troops defeated the French. • Played a key role in the founding of Haiti.
Why did U.S. leaders become suspicious?	• Napoleon once again owned Louisiana and knew that French could block the westward growth of the U.S. and could block trade and that French could control trade along the Mississippi River.
Why did Napoleon sell Louisiana to the U.S.?	• He needed money for the war that was about to start with Great Britain; French had no troops in Louisiana. • Instead of territory Napoleon wanted money for supplies. Napoleon realized that if the U.S. owned Louisiana, the U.S. could challenge Great Britain's power in North America. • Ambassador bought Louisiana from France for $15 million dollars and signed a treaty of purchase on May 2, 1803. • Size of the U.S. almost doubled as a result.

FIGURE 4.9. History notes in two-column format.

strategy enables students to think through and map out their arguments before writing (see Figure 4.12). Students with top-down styles may prefer to brainstorm their two or three main reasons first; bottom-up thinkers may prefer to start by brainstorming details and then comparing those in order to label them with category names, which in turn become the two or three main ideas they use to support their thesis.

Narrative Information

ELEMENTARY SCHOOL

Just as it is important for students to learn the way language is organized in expository contexts, it is also necessary for them to learn how narrative information is organized so that they can successfully read literature, retell a story, and write their own narratives. Students can first learn to recognize the common elements in every story and then use their knowledge to evaluate other narratives. Teachers can then foster students' application of this knowledge to reading comprehension and writing, using scaffolding and explicit organizational strategies. Specifically, knowledge of story grammar assists students in planning and writing their own stories by providing them with a strategic way to brainstorm and organize the content before writing (Graham & Harris, 2005).

Making the instruction more concrete and "hands-on" will provide additional support for students who struggle with language expression. Story Grammar Marker (see Moreau & Fidrych-Puzzo, 2002), utilizes a hands-on approach that students can use to learn and apply the essential elements of a story. The symbols cue students to include the important narrative features: characters, setting, "kick-off" (initiating action), character's big problem, character's feelings about the big problem, main solution (links back to big problem), steps to the solution, and character's feelings about the solution. Students can use these prompts when they

Triple Note Tote: A three-column chart that helps you organize information you need to know.

When: Helpful when taking notes from a textbook or reviewing terms or information you need to know for a test.

How:
1. Write the main idea, question, or term in the first column.

Question/Term	Answer/Definition	Strategy
What are the steps of photosynthesis?		

2. Write the details, answer, or definition in the second column.

Question/Term	Answer/Definition	Strategy
What are the steps of photosynthesis?	1. Water and nutrients are transported from the roots, up the stem (xylem) to the leaves. 2. Light from the sun shines on leaves, and light energy is trapped by chlorophyll and stored. 3. Energy trapped by the chlorophyll turns carbon dioxide from air into sugars and releases oxygen into air. 4. Sugars are transported down the step (phloem) to be stored in other parts of the plant. Cell uses this food to grow.	

FIGURE 4.10. Sample of a Triple Note Tote. The chart itself is from ResearchILD and FableVision (2003). Copyright 2003 by ResearchILD. Reprinted by permission.

Sometimes people need someone to convince them.

Strong leaders like Martin Luther King can change the world. Leaders can organize and direct people.	People are perfectly capable of forming their own ideas. People don't need a leader.
MLK Attorneys convincing a jury	Hitler was a convincing leader, but he led the world to a terrible war.
Social studies textbook Class discussion	Social Studies, Chapter 11.

Sometimes people need a leader; however, people should be cautious and ask a lot of questions, because leaders can lead you in the wrong direction.

FIGURE 4.11. Sample completed PROVE template. The template itself is from Scanlon (2002). Copyright 2002 by David Scanlon. Reprinted by permission.

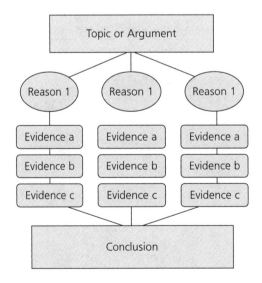

FIGURE 4.12. The Pieces of a Thesis strategy for organizing analytical writing.

are orally retelling, writing a summary of a story, or generating their own narrative. Teachers can also provide graphic organizers that include the important elements of a narrative for students to use during prewriting activities. Prompts can be faded as students internalize the structure.

MIDDLE AND HIGH SCHOOL

Teachers can revisit the structure of a narrative at the upper grades and adapt narrative organizers to include more sophisticated analyses of the material. Students can plot out elements of assigned literature for use in small-group and whole-class discussions, and for summarizing what they have read.

Students at the upper levels can extend the foundational knowledge of sorting and categorizing they have acquired in the early grades to organize elements in literature. For example, students can track character traits when reading novels, and can use that information to identify themes in character development across literature and to predict actions of characters in new novels they are reading (see Appendix 6 for a blank Character Traits Sheet).

CONCLUSION

"A place for everything and everything in its place" is an age-old saying that is still highly relevant to our daily lives. Given the wealth of information that students process daily, and the multiple demands placed on their time by homework, extracurricular activities, and hobbies, it is evident that an efficient mental "filing system" is essential for their success in school. Such a filing system will ensure that information is grouped and stored in the most meaningful and efficient manner, so that students can retrieve what they need when they need it; the information will also be laid out in a manner that promotes critical thinking skills.

CHAPTER 5

Remembering

Teaching Students How to Retain
and Mentally Manipulate Information

DONNA M. KINCAID and NANCY TRAUTMAN

> Memory . . . is the diary that we all carry about with us.
> —OSCAR WILDE

Memory is a record of our experience, and so learning is dependent on memory. To learn, students must receive, store, retain, and retrieve information on demand. As students develop and gain experience, they continually add to their reserves of memories and new information. Students learn and remember through direct experiences—that is, what they have seen, felt, heard, or touched. In addition, they acquire information through indirect experiences with text, visual data, images, verbal narratives, and emotional experiences. The accumulated information and experiences that are gathered into memory, either deliberately or by indirect means, shape the responses and choices that students make (Sprenger, 1999; Swanson & Sáez, 2003). Without the accumulated memory of these experiences, it would not be possible for students to learn; they would repeat the same actions, whether right or wrong, again and again.

In this chapter, we provide an overview of the major memory processes with a focus on the central role of working memory. We also describe *why* memory is so important for learning and discuss *how* students employ strategies to make their memories more durable and improve their academic performance. We discuss specific metacognitive strategies that can be taught in the classroom to improve students' ability to retain needed information, retrieve facts on demand, manipulate information mentally, recall processes or concepts, and ultimately learn. Some of the strategies presented in this chapter have been validated in controlled studies; others are based on research in classrooms; and many have been used effectively in the educational therapy setting.

WHY IS MEMORY SO IMPORTANT FOR THE LEARNING PROCESS?

Students are often frustrated by the volume of information that they are expected to juggle and access mentally. Beginning in preschool, students must rely on memory in order to learn. Social rules in school are learned through both explicit instruction and direct experiences. The guidelines for these school-based behaviors must be remembered. In preschool, students also begin to learn basic academic skills. Among the first academic skills that student must learn are the relationships between the letters and their accompanying sounds, and between the numerals and the quantities they represent. In addition, new processes, such as the left-to-right reading and writing patterns in English and other Western languages, must be learned. The foundational information that young students learn in the early grades becomes the basis for their higher-level thinking and their increasingly sophisticated analysis and problem solving. As students go on to middle and high school, they are also become responsible for remembering procedural information that is important for their academic performance, such as daily and weekly schedules, assignments for multiple classes, materials needed, and procedures to be followed (Hughes, 1996). Thus memory, in general, and working memory, in particular, are essential for students to function successfully in school.

Memory is inconsistent and variable, both from one student to another and from one task to the next for the same student. For example, some students are able to learn and remember the multiplication tables without effort, while others practice diligently but still struggle with recall. An individual student may be able to recall and retrieve the entire roster of a favorite baseball team or musical group, but may not be able to remember the names of the three types of rocks for the science quiz. Memory weaknesses are often associated with learning disabilities, and may affect students' retrieval of meaningful or nonmeaningful information, ability to hold and manipulate information mentally, or automatic retrieval of information from long-term memory (Mastropieri & Scruggs, 1998; Swanson & Saez, 2003).

The ability to learn depends on a student's ability to incorporate new information into an existing schema or mental framework in order to create a lasting memory. The role played by directed attention and strategy use in this process is crucial for all learners (Torgesen, 1996). Thus, teachers and students who develop a strategic mindset toward memory tasks will be able to develop a repertoire of executive function strategies that help them to learn and remember new information and achieve academic success.

Basic Memory Types and Functions

An understanding of basic memory processes is useful for teachers who seek to help their students develop executive function strategies that will improve their ability to remember and retrieve needed information. Human memory is a highly complex system for information processing, storage, and retrieval. Within this sys-

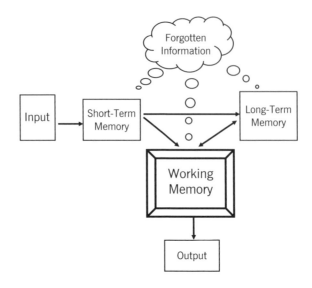

FIGURE 5.1. Simplified schematic of the central role of working memory.

tem, there are three general types of memory: *short-term memory, working memory,* and *long-term memory* (Baddeley, 2006; Torgesen, 1996). Figure 5.1 illustrates these three memory processes and the relationships among them. In addition, *automatic memory* facilitates function by helping students to access well-known or rote information rapidly (Swanson & Sachse-Lee, 2003). These memory processes are closely interconnected, yet each contributes to learning in a slightly different way. While working memory is regarded as the most important executive function process, all aspects of memory interact closely with these executive function processes, as will be discussed in this chapter.

Short-Term Memory: Gateway to Learning

All information that is received through the senses—that is, everything that we see, hear, feel, smell, and touch—is perceived, processed, and placed in short-term memory. Short-term memory holds a limited amount of information (on average, seven "bits" of information) for a limited amount of time (a few seconds) while it is processed (Goldman-Rakic, 1992). The brain constantly monitors and filters the sensory input it receives in the short-term memory and categorizes the incoming information into "discard," "use right away," and "long-term storage" categories, much as incoming mail may be quickly sorted into "junk mail," "look at right away," and "will need this later" piles.

Information that is not recognized as important is immediately discarded and lost. Most of the vast amounts of sensory input that the brain receives are not committed to memory beyond this initial receptive interval (Torgesen, 1996). The fate of the sensory input, or information that is received, is often determined by the level of attention: Students who are able to direct and sustain their attention are more likely to retain needed information (Tannock, 2008). For example, a student who hears the teacher announce, "There will be a class party this week," is very likely to "tune in" and attend to the next piece of information, "The end-of-semester pizza lunch is on Friday." On the other hand, when attention is not engaged, a student may find that he or she has no recall of the announcement and may miss important assignments, as well as the pizza party. Thus selective attention plays a critical role in how information is processed in short-term memory. The conscious effort to attend to information represents the role of executive function processes in attention and learning. Information that is recognized as important stands out for the individual and enters the working memory system, where it may be used right away or eventually be encoded into long-term memory and retained (Tannock, 2008).

Working Memory: The Mind's Scratchpad

Working memory is an active and limited-capacity memory system that acquires information from short- or long-term memory, sensory input, and/or automatic memory, and then holds the information for a short time while a task is being performed (Baddeley, 2006). Thus it is an intermediary system that has an enormous impact on academic performance. Working memory is proposed to be the central cognitive control process that focuses the mind, directs mental efforts, accomplishes tasks, and ignores distractions (de Fockert, Rees, Frith, & Lavie, 2001; Swanson, 1999; Tannock, 2008). In fact, it is argued that working memory functions as the central executive that directs all other cognitive processes, including inhibition of impulses, shifting attention, and directing effort (Baddeley, 2006; Swanson & Șaez, 2003). It has also been proposed that working memory can be compared to a scratchpad or desktop—a neurological workstation where current stimuli and tasks are placed "up front" and managed (Daneman & Carpenter, 1980). Within this model, there are two pathways: Visual information is processed on a *visual–spatial sketchpad*, and auditory information is held and rehearsed on a *phonological loop* (Baddeley, 2006). Working memory enables students to hold auditory, written, or visual information in mind long enough to understand a sequence of words and ideas, and also allows students to retain facts so that they can be formulated into expressive language in the form of verbal statements, written sentences, or coherent paragraphs. Working memory weaknesses, therefore, have a significant impact on academic performance.

Activities that place large amounts of other tasks or stressors on a student's "desktop" may cause inefficiencies or breakdown in the system (Baddeley, 2006). For example, tasks requiring students to retain large amounts of information in their working memory while simultaneously manipulating information—such as remembering the steps for solving a complex math problem, remembering the characters in a narrative, or writing an essay—require a large amount of cognitive effort that competes for processing space with other mental functions. If the cognitive demands of retaining the information are too great, these demands may diminish the mental resources that are available to perform higher-level reasoning tasks such as analysis or synthesis (Gathercole, Lamont, & Alloway, 2006). In addition, external distractions or emotional stressors tax the central executive system and impair students' ability to attend to learning, inhibit impulses, and persevere (Baddeley, 2006). The role of emotion in executive function is discussed in greater detail in Chapter 8.

Working memory thus plays a critical role in listening comprehension, reading comprehension, oral communication, written expression, math problem solving, and efficient task completion. Clearly, efficient working memory is critical for successful academic performance and long-term learning. Academic tasks that require the integration and coordination of multiple subskills usually rely heavily on working memory and include the following:

- *Completing tasks*—remembering the steps of a procedure, the requirements of an assignment, or a set of verbal directions.
- *Reading comprehension*—remembering characters, events and details, sequences of ideas, and elements of plot.
- *Written language*—simultaneously accessing the spelling of a word, the words in a sentence, and the organization of a paragraph or short answer during the writing process.
- *Math*—mental computation and problem solving, carrying numbers during the division process, regrouping when multiplying, and remembering answers to steps during multistep problem solving.
- *Note taking*—simultaneously retaining ideas and organizing information while formulating notes.
- *Following directions*—remembering detailed directions while performing other tasks.
- *Responding to oral questions in class*—recalling all parts of a question or a response while waiting to answer.

Automatic Memory

Automatic memory is a component of the brain's retrieval system that enables a person to retrieve familiar or known facts rapidly from long-term memory when they are needed for problem solving. When automatic memory works efficiently, it activates information and can quickly supply working memory with the information needed on the desktop for problem solving. This relieves working memory of the need to perform these functions and thus frees it for higher-level problem-solving tasks, such as comprehension, analysis, synthesis, mathematical problem solving, and complex writing (Swanson & Sachse-Lee, 2001). For example, when the sounds of letters are retrieved automatically for decoding, automatic memory has rapidly processed the images of individual letters, combinations of letters, word parts, whole words, or frequently occurring phrases and has matched them with their sounds and meanings, which is a critical process in reading fluency (Shaywitz, 2003). Automatic memory also supports accurate spelling, as the spelling patterns for many words can be written without conscious cognitive effort. Similarly, rapid automatic recall of math facts enables students to devote cognitive effort to the reasoning involved in analyzing and solving complex math problems.

Academic tasks that require automatic memory include the following:

- Rapid recall of answers to basic addition, subtraction, multiplication, and division problems.
- Rapid naming of colors, numerals, and letters.
- Rapid recognition of letters and phonemes.
- Rapid reading of sight words, such as *an, the*, and *who.*
- Rapid retrieval of spelling patterns.

Long-Term Memory

Long-term memory cements information that can be used over hours, days, or a lifetime. It has been thought of as an almost permanent storage system with unlimited capacity (Hughes, 1996). Individuals store information—that is, words, images, themes, or ideas—according to complex neurological associations that are created within the brain's filing system. These associations, which enable retrieval of information, involve a rich variety of pathways that are established as the information is encoded and stored. Associations may be kinetic, visual, verbal, sensory, emotional, or abstract; they may be created passively (i.e., without conscious cognitive effort), or they may be developed metacognitively through the use of intentional executive function strategies (Mastropieri & Scruggs, 1991). Attention and strategy use are thus critical for the retrieval of information in long-term memory.

Academic tasks that require long-term memory include the following:

- *General*—learning of curriculum content.
- *Math*—remembering algorithms for computation.
- *Oral language*—retrieving ideas and information, developing vocabulary knowledge.
- *Written language*—recalling ideas and information.
- *Reading comprehension*—recalling plots, events, character traits.

HOW CAN WE TEACH STUDENTS STRATEGIES TO IMPROVE THEIR MEMORY?

The model for day-to-day classroom teaching of executive function strategies provided in Chapter 2 suggests that teachers sequence instruction in memory strategies as follows. First, it is important that students understand each strategy, why it aids memory, and when they can apply it. Students should then be explicitly taught how to use the strategy; thus direct instruction and teacher modeling of strategy use are critical. Finally, students should be asked to use a specific strategy for a task, and should then be required to reflect on how it worked for them. Later in this chapter, we present a variety of executive function strategies that can facilitate students' ability to remember and learn needed information. In general, such strategies are based on four basic approaches, which we discuss below:

1. Attending to details
2. Repetition, rehearsal, and review
3. Attaching meaning
4. Chunking information

Attending to Details

The role of attention is so important that some researchers contend that without attention, there is virtually no memory (de Fockert et al., 2001). The process of focusing attention is especially important for efficient working memory. The brain's ability to make connections, retain information, and retrieve it is enhanced by heightened attention (Tannock, 2008). If information is not marked as important or relevant by the brain, most of it will enter short-term memory very briefly and then be dismissed before it can be committed to long-term memory (Torgesen, 1996). Heightened attention makes information, experiences, or processes "stand out" in the brain, and is the vital first step in separating relevant information from other sensory input. The brain benefits from a signal, either external or internal, to prompt it to focus when something important is coming. For example, verbal cues such as "Your homework for the night is . . . " or "The three key factors in the decision to engage in the Civil War were . . . " enhance attention. Visual cues—such as colors (red, yellow) that signal danger, bold letters, animated displays, and startling images—all prompt heightened attention and contribute to our ability to remember.

Sustaining the attention necessary for effective information processing in a classroom setting or during study times is difficult for many students. Their attention may be easily diverted by external factors, such as other students, activities, or noises in the vicinity. Internal distractions may be equally disruptive to a student's sustained attention. Students who are preoccupied with the anticipation of an upcoming event, the processing of a past event, or the workings of their imagination cannot easily attend, and therefore cannot easily remember information. All students, and particularly those with learning differences, benefit from developing greater awareness of the role that attention plays in memory, and from learning executive function strategies to improve their ability to direct and sustain their focus on instruction and material (Swanson, Hoskyn, & Lee, 1999).

Repetition, Rehearsal, and Review

The "three R's" of memory are repetition, rehearsal, and review. To cement a small amount of information in memory, it may be helpful to "visit" it again—that is, to repeat, rehearse, and review the information (Baddeley, 2006). Verbal rehearsal of needed information can provide an auditory stimulus when students hear themselves repeat the information. Copying material over may also be helpful, as the combined effects of the visual focus of reading and the motor rehearsal of writing engage both the visual and kinesthetic modalities and make the rehearsal more effective. Rehearsal may emphasize primarily visual pathways as well. For example, students may develop visual images when they read texts or novels. The transfer of print to words and words to images requires the student to create and rehearse cognitive connections, and thus can improve both memory and comprehension (Bell, 1986). Repetition may also involve kinesthetic rehearsal; for example, students can tap on numerals to reinforce their learning of addition facts. Students will benefit from awareness of the rehearsal modality or modalities that are most effective for them—visual, auditory, kinesthetic, and/or tactile—and the development of strategies that capitalize on their unique strengths.

Attaching Meaning

Attaching meaning to new information is a powerful memory tool. A framework, or background knowledge, is important for learning: It provides the student with cognitive associations that make it easier for the student to incorporate, comprehend, and retrieve the new information. Understanding and remembering new information is thus often facilitated by a comparison to something familiar and known. For example, to describe an unusual landscape, you might compare it to a known landscape or image. You might say that the beaches of Bermuda look like Cape Cod, but with sand that is pink and plants that have large shiny leaves and profuse flowers. That comparison would provide a preexisting knowledge base (for those who have visited Cape Cod) with which to link the new information. Overall, a student's knowledge base is a valuable foundation that helps him or her to perform higher-level problem solving—that is, to understand, evaluate, compare, analyze, and think abstractly about new information (Sprenger, 1999; Swanson et al., 1999).

Information that students need to learn can be given additional meaning by intentionally creating associations with a student's preexisting background knowledge or by using verbal and visual associations, acronyms, acrostics, or rhymes to make it meaningful. Timelines, information maps, webs, and charts also help students to organize information and create associations (Mastropieri & Scruggs, 1991). Attaching meaning to information via these strategies creates a more complex system of cognitive connections or pathways, which improves the brain's ability to locate and retrieve information from long-term memory when needed (Swanson et al., 1999).

Chunking Information

Chunking information, or the process of combining ideas or items into fewer units, helps students to store and retrieve information (Swanson et al., 1999). These groupings can be verbal or visual, and may be based on sequential blocks of information or a variety of categorical groups (e.g., oceans or battles of the Civil War). For example, a student might learn pi by grouping it into sets of three digits, or might rely on a visual image of the outline of a word to recall the numbers. The numbers that people need to remember are often pregrouped to take advantage of the brain's preference for chunked information. Phone numbers in North America, for example, are easier to recall because they are grouped into a three-digit area code, a three-digit prefix, and a four-digit locator number. U.S. Social Security numbers are also chunked for more efficient recall. In school, multiplication tables can be made easier to recall by grouping them into patterns and categories, according to their products. Similarly, the periodic table in chemistry organizes 111 elements into logical patterns according to their physical and chemical properties and provides the organization of a visual grid. Chunking or grouping information is a highly effective memory strategy, as this makes it possible to remember more "bits" of information than the human brain could remember if the information were encoded individually (Mastropieri & Scruggs, 1991).

WHAT EXECUTIVE FUNCTION STRATEGIES CAN BE TAUGHT TO HELP STUDENTS REMEMBER NEEDED INFORMATION IN SCHOOL?

In the remainder of this chapter, we describe specific strategies within each of the core curriculum areas, as well as strategies for studying and test taking. The majority of the strategies have been effective in clinical research studies (conducted by ResearchILD) in public school settings and in individual educational therapy sessions, but have not yet been experimentally validated. These strategies, which incorporate the key elements for improving memory (attention to details, repetition/rehearsal/review, attaching meaning, and chunking information) accommodate different learning styles and can easily be adapted across the grades.

Research has shown that the use of *mnemonics* is among the most effective methods for improving students' memory for factual information (Mastropieri & Scruggs, 1991, 1998; Scruggs & Mastropieri, 2000). Mnemonics are memory-enhancing strategies that help students to remember essential steps or important information. The word *mnemonic* literally means "aids memory." In practice, mnemonics enable students to make new information and associate that information with what they already know" (Eggen & Kauchak, 1992). In addition, mnemonics help to "recode, transform, or elaborate information by making meaningful connections to seemingly unconnected information" (Carney, Levin, & Levin, 1993). When students are able to make such meaningful associations, they achieve greater success with transfer of this information into long-term memory and later retrieval (Mastropieri & Scruggs, 1998). Because students with learning and attention difficulties often do not create meaningful links on their own, they may need direct, systematic instruction in when and how to use memory strategies.

Many different types of mnemonics have proven to be successful in improving retention of information among all learners, and specifically among students with learning difficulties (Mastropieri & Scruggs, 1991, 1998; Scruggs & Mastropieri, 2000). These include key words, peg words, acronyms, acrostics, and visuals. Most people have heard of or used mnemonics at different times in their lives, such as "HOMES," an acronym for remembering the Great Lakes (Huron, Ontario, Michigan, Erie, and Superior), and "Every Good Boy Does Fine," an acrostic for remembering the notes on the lines of the treble clef on a musical staff (EGBDF). Often different types of mnemonic strategies are used together. For instance, an acoustic link (word) can be paired with a visual image (picture), as in the keyword method, to further solidify the information in memory and thereby to increase students' ability to store and retrieve the information (Mastropieri & Scruggs, 1998).

The use of *crazy phrases* from BrainCogs (ResearchILD & FableVision, 2003) is another example of an effective strategy for memorizing sequential information. As discussed in Chapters 1 and 2, in order for strategy instruction to be effective, students need to know *what* the strategy is, and *when* and *how* the strategy can be used. A example of how to teach the crazy phrases strategy to students is provided below. (Specific examples of crazy phrases are provided later in this chapter, and a template for teaching students how to create crazy phrases can be found in Appendix 7.)

> *What*: A *crazy phrase* is a made-up wacky phrase or sentence to help you remember particular information in a specific order.
>
> *When*: Crazy phrases are helpful when you need to remember names, places, events, or operations in a specific order (e.g., planets in the solar system, countries on a map, steps in long division).
>
> *How*: Use a crazy phrase to remember the steps of the strategy itself: "Lizards Wrestle Crunchy Pretzels."
>
> - List the information in order.
> - Write the first letter from each word.
> - Create a silly sentence whose words begin with these letters. Try to make up a sentence that creates a funny picture in your head.
> - Practice the sentence until you remember it easily.

Students' profiles of strengths and weaknesses often influence their selection of different strategies. Some students prefer the use of visual strategies, such as cartoons, graphic organizers, and templates. Mnemonics are often embedded within these organizers to enhance their effectiveness. For those who prefer verbal or auditory strategies, chants, rhymes, and songs work well. Whatever memory strategies are used, it is essential to give students time to practice and rehearse each strategy or mnemonic, for "a strategy that cannot be recalled, cannot be used" (Harris et al., 2008, p. 18). As students learn and practice memory strategies that are modeled by their teachers, many often create strategies of their own that match their individual learning styles; other students prefer and benefit from teacher-created mnemonics.

Like other executive function strategies, memory strategies can be taught explicitly in the classroom to help all students learn and perform more successfully. It is important for teachers to start by trying only a few strategies with their students. As students experience success with these strategies, they can add other memory strategies to their repertoires. Research does not specify an optimal number of mnemonics that can be successfully taught at any given time. Variability in how much information students can learn mnemonically depends on many factors, including the difficulty of the content, the students' ages and abilities, the meaningfulness of the mnemonic associations, and the extent to which the strategies are rehearsed. Research with students who have learning difficulties suggests that mnemonic instruction does not inhibit such students' learning by drawing their attention away from the main content; rather, it enhances their learning (Mastropieri, Sweda, & Scruggs, 2000). Nonetheless, teachers should be careful to select high-priority and difficult terms from a unit, and to allow students sufficient time to practice using memory strategies systematically. In this way, students learn what is *most important* to remember from an area of study, and their working memory systems are not overloaded. Specific strategies for use in different areas within the school curriculum are provided below.

Memory Strategies for Reading Comprehension

Reading comprehension is a complex process. The difference between skilled readers and those who struggle with reading is often due in large part to working memory deficits (Swanson, 2000). Many students experience frustration at not being able to recall key characters, events, and story details. Students may pass over unfamiliar vocabulary words for fear that they will lose their place or forget the rest of the story. In addition, they may not make the connection that particular words are important to the larger context. Nonfluent readers who have underlying weaknesses with the decoding process or with automatic memory read slowly. In doing so, they often forget key information as they read. These readers expend so much of their attention on the reading process that they have difficulty under-

TABLE 5.1. Memory Strategies for Reading Comprehension

Type of reading material	Strategy	Purpose
Fiction/nonfiction	STAR strategy	To identify main ideas, using the five W's and memory strategies
Fiction	Chapter summary organizer	To record specific information about chapters and write chapter summaries
Fiction	Title and Why	To record the most important feature of each chapter
Fiction/nonfiction	Book notes (margin notes, Post-it Notes, text codes)	To record information directly in a book or on removable Post-its; advance questions or organizers help direct the reading process

standing what they read. Nonfiction text is sometimes even more difficult than fiction, as many students struggle to organize information in a way that helps them to understand and remember the main ideas and the details on both a short-term and a long-term basis.

Strengthening working memory capacity through strategy instruction allows students to engage effectively in more complex cognitive processes, such as reading comprehension (McNamara & Scott, 2001). Across the grades, students can learn to use strategies to help them remember important information as they read different types of text. The *active reading* strategies described below and summarized in Table 5.1 heighten students' attention to important information and show them how to make meaningful connections as they read. As they attach meaning to smaller pieces of information and create visual and other aids to record important information, students' memory capacity is enhanced.

The STAR Strategy

The STAR strategy (Meltzer et al., 2006), introduced in Chapter 1, is a multipurpose strategy that helps students to organize, remember, and study information. This strategy can be adapted for use in different content areas, at different grade levels, and with texts of varying levels of complexity. The key elements of *who, what, when, where,* and *why* (the "five W's") focus students' attention on the main ideas and supporting details; the complexity of the format shifts as the complexity of the information increases. For younger students or those with learning disabilities, an organizer in the shape of an actual star can be used (see Figures 1.15a and 1.15b in Chapter 1 for examples); for older students, the key elements of the STAR strategy can be formatted in a linear design, for use with increasingly sophisticated content information (see Figure 5.2). As students actively read both fiction and nonfiction, the STAR chart helps them to stop, reflect, and record key information, thereby enhancing their memory of important facts. An additional column is incorporated

Term	WHO?	WHAT did it do?	WHEN?	WHERE?	WHY is it important?	STRATEGY to remember
Proclamation of 1763	Signed by King George III	Stopped English settlement west of Appalachian Mountains; required those already there to return east	1763	England/ Colonies	Attempt to ease tensions with Native Americans	
Sugar Act	Passed by English Parliament	Increased taxes on imported sugar and other items; doubled taxes on foreign goods from England; forbade import of foreign rum and French wine	1764	England/ Colonies	To decrease the war debt from the French and Indian War and help pay for running the colonies	
Currency Act	Affected colonies	Prohibited colonists from issuing any paper money	1764	Colonies	Bad for economy of colonies in North and South; colonists were against it	
Stamp Act	Passed by English Parliament	First direct tax on American colonies; taxed all printed materials	1765	America	To pay for military organization in America; Americans paid taxes not only to local government but also directly to England; colonists united in opposition	In 1765, the Stamp Act was alive!
Sons of Liberty	Members from colonial towns	Underground organization opposed to Stamp Act	1765	America— number of colonial towns	Used violence to force British stamp agents to resign and stopped many American merchants from ordering British goods	

Drive to Thrive © ResearchILD 2004

FIGURE 5.2. Example of the Star Strategy: The Revolutionary War.

in the chart shown in Figure 5.2, to prompt students as they study the material to create a memory strategy that helps them mentally manipulate and retrieve the critical themes and details.

Chapter Summary Organizers

Chapter summary organizers are used to formally document key information from a chapter, helping students to narrow down the most important elements for a summary statement. Maintaining a summary record of main ideas helps students to stop, reflect, and recall specific events and character details for class discussions and related assignments, including those that require specific examples and quotes. This strategy is most effective for elementary and middle school students. A reproducible Chapter Summary Organizer is provided as Appendix 8.

Title and Why

Title and Why is another ResearchILD strategy that we have used to help students recall specific information as they read chapter books or novels. Similar to a chapter summary organizer, this strategy prompts a student to stop, reflect, and write. Here students recall the most important feature of each chapter and record it directly in the book or on a Post-it Note. If chapters already have a title, students rename the chapter in their own words and write. If the chapter does not have a title, students first create a title that conveys the main idea. After students have read a novel, these chapter summaries are effective memory joggers and allow them to retrieve specific ideas and details more efficiently. As this active reading strategy requires a minimal amount of writing, it may be especially effective for students who struggle with written expression, such as those with dysgraphia.

Book Notes

Book Notes are useful in various forms. Many students with working memory difficulties benefit from writing directly in their own copy of a book, using such strategies as margin notes and text codes. It is helpful for teachers to identify what students should look for, think about, and record during the reading process; this will help students to focus their attention on critical information. When writing in a book is not an option, the versatility of Post-it Notes makes them excellent tools for recording information. These notes help students to memorize major themes and details for class discussions and writing assignments.

Memory Strategies for Written Language

Memory strategies for written language are summarized in Table 5.2 and described below.

TABLE 5.2. Memory Strategies for Written Language

Writing focus	Strategy	Purpose
Writing sentences or paragraphs	Brainstorm words and phrases in advance	To recall key words or phrases for sentence or paragraph writing
Writing paragraphs or essays	BOTEC from Essay Express	Mnemonic to aid recall of steps in the writing process
	Pieces of a Thesis	Use of courtroom scene analogy to write a persuasive essay
	PROVE (Scanlon, 2002)	An acronym to remember steps for presenting facts and supporting evidence
Transitions within and between paragraphs	Lists or charts of common transition words/phrases and their uses	To recall the words that improve the flow of writing
Sentence starters	Lists of sentence starters	To help students who "get stuck" during the writing process and need help remembering how to begin the next sentence
Editing	SPORTS	To recall what to look for during the editing process
Note taking	Partially completed outline	To provide structured format for note taking; to give conceptual framework for unit of study
	Color highlighting Fonts sizes	To visually differentiate main ideas, details, key vocabulary

Note. See text for explanations for acronyms.

Memory Strategies for Formulating Essays

Writing is a highly complex process. "The effective writer must negotiate the rules and mechanics of writing while maintaining a focus on factors such as organization, form and features, purposes and goals, audience needs and perspectives, and evaluation of the communication between author and reader" (Harris et al., 2008, p. 3). Students can experience difficulty with one or more of these elements; in particular, students with poor working memory may struggle with many aspects of the writing process. These particular students often have excellent ideas, but they may struggle to retain their ideas or the central theme as they formulate words, sentences, paragraphs, and essays, resulting in inefficient work or poor written performance (McNamara & Scott, 2001). These students may also struggle to remember all the components of the writing process, and this may make essay writing even more difficult. Demands on working memory can be reduced by activating students' knowledge and brainstorming keywords and phrases with them before they write sentences or paragraphs. Students can then use their brainstorming lists to formulate sentences. In addition, easy access to strategies and tools (e.g., writing templates, sentence starters) can improve the quality of students' essays.

BOTEC FROM ESSAY EXPRESS

Essay Express (ResearchILD & FableVision, 2005), discussed in Chapter 2, is an interactive software program that teaches a systematic approach to the writing process, which is essential when middle and high school students are writing essays. A strategy from Essay Express is the BOTEC an acronym for (Brainstorm, Organize, Topic sentence, Evidence, and Conclusion) that helps students to remember the steps and procedures in the writing process. (See Chapter 2 for a fuller discussion of BOTEC.)

PIECES OF A THESIS

Pieces of a Thesis (see Chapter 4, specifically Figure 4.12) is a strategy for organizing and developing a persuasive essay. The analogy of a courtroom scene can be used as a basis to help students remember to:

- State an *argument*.
- State the *reasons* for making this argument.
- Begin with an (*opening statement*).
- Provide *specific evidence*.
- End with a *concluding statement*.

PROVE

PROVE (Scanlon, 2002) is an acronym that is designed to help students recall the five steps involved in presenting factual information and supporting explanations. The PROVE strategy (see Chapter 4) guides students to:

- Present information to be proved.
- Reveal information to support that knowledge.
- Offer examples or explanations to support that knowledge.
- Verify knowledge, using examples or challenges.
- Express knowledge in a summary statement.

LISTS OR CHARTS OF TRANSITION WORDS/PHRASES

Lists or charts of common transitions are useful for students who are able to write basic sentences, but have difficulty remembering to use effective signals to help their ideas flow smoothly. Categorizing signal words and phrases according to their use is helpful, so that students can choose words or phrases that indicate order (*first, second*), additions (*also, furthermore*), comparison and contrast (*although, however*), cause and effect (*therefore, as a result*), and conclusions (*in summary, as you can see*).

SENTENCE STARTERS

Sentence starters are helpful for students who have difficulty getting started or who "get stuck" in the process of paragraph or essay writing. These prompts help students to feel less reliant on memory and allow them to proceed with the flow of their ideas. Their sentences can be edited in the final stage of writing if necessary. Teachers can initially provide students with lists, which they can later personalize and adapt to fit their writing style. Some examples from Essay Express are listed below.

One of the most remarkable . . .	Another significant event . . .
The most significant . . .	Another important factor . . .
The primary reason . . .	Another possible explanation . . .
One of the most important . . .	Another factor to consider . . .

THE ISA STRATEGY

ISA is an acronym for a three-step strategy for embedding quotes into an essay or paper. It helps students who cannot remember this procedure from one writing assignment to the next. ISA guides students to:

Introduce:
- State who said something.
- Indicate when it was said and in what scene.

State:
- Copy the quote exactly; stick to short quotes.
- Use parenthetical citations.
- Use " . . . " for skipped words.

Analyze—the hardest part:
- How does this quote support your thesis?
- If it doesn't work, change the quote or your thesis!

Memory Strategies for Editing

Editing checklists are useful for students of all grade levels, and many are presented in Chapter 7. Mnemonics, such as the one presented below, can help students to remember the particular steps for checking written work.

SPORTS (Meltzer et al., 2006) is an acronym for items in an expanded checklist that is useful for middle and high school students. A visual image, such as sports equipment, a basketball hoop, or a goalpost, helps trigger the memory of the acronym for visual learners. Students *score* by using the mnemonic to edit their written work properly.

SPORTS
Sentence structure
Punctuation
Organization
Repetition
Tenses
Spelling

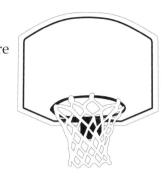

Memory Strategies for Note Taking

Note taking is especially challenging for students with poor working memory who have difficulty with multitasking; for example, they struggle to listen to the teacher at the same time as they process the information and formulate notes. These multistep processes become even more challenging when new information is presented. Research suggests a correlation between handwriting (orthographic coding) and working memory capacity in relation to the quality and quantity of notes written (Baerveldt, Madison, & Martinussen, 2008). In other words, students with working memory difficulties may write fewer and less detailed notes. The same working memory difficulties affect students' ability to take notes from text: Students may read, focusing on the material, yet may not actively engage in the process by stopping to ask questions and take notes. In the end, students' recall of important information may suffer, and they may have to reread the material repeatedly in order to remember key information. The following strategies are effective in helping students become more effective note takers with better ability to recall the content.

  • *Partial outlines (or note-taking templates)* provide students with organizational schemas for taking notes. These outlines lessen the amount of writing required by students, thereby decreasing the working memory demands and allowing students to focus on the main ideas. Furthermore, these organizational schemas help students to conceptualize the "big picture" and enhance their understanding and later recall of the content as they take notes.
  • *Color highlighting* helps students to separate the themes from the details and to memorize the information more easily. Teachers can teach this strategy to their entire class and have students use the strategy as a consistent part of their note-taking process. The colors chosen for various aspects of note taking should be used consistently. For instance, green can be used for the main ideas, blue for the details, and yellow for key vocabulary.
  • *Different-size letters or different fonts* can also be used to help students to differentiate the main ideas from the details, as in this example:

Four Major Food Groups

Dairy

Meat

Fruits/vegetables

Grains

Memory Strategies for Math Computation and Reasoning

Memory strategies for math computation and reasoning as summarized in Table 5.3 and described below.

Memory Strategies for Math Fact Fluency

Many students struggle with the automatic retrieval of math facts and procedures, although their math reasoning and problem-solving abilities are strong. Specific strategies can be taught to help students to recall math facts more efficiently. Creating rhymes and crazy phrases, making associations with what they already know, using verbal and visual mnemonics, and incorporating kinesthetic movements can all help to improve students' math automaticity. Whatever strategies are used, frequent opportunities for repetition and practice are essential for students to improve their recall of math facts.

TABLE 5.3. Memory Strategies for Math Computation and Reasoning

Math focus area	Strategy	Purpose
Fact fluency	Rhymes Visual representations Visual–kinesthetic strategies Crazy phrases	To help students recall basic math facts more efficiently
Formulae/procedures	Songs Stories Acronyms FOIL and Face Strategy notebooks	To help students remember procedural steps and formulae; to provide quick references for students to use when completing math problems
Word problems	Underline direction words, number the steps in the problem, underline the question (color highlighting may also be used)	To focus attention on what to do, the number of steps involved in the problem, and the question to be solved
	CUPS KNOW RAPS	Acronyms to help students recall key steps to solve word problems
Checking	POUNCE	An acronym to help students remember to check their work when done

Note. See text for explanations of acronyms. For more details regarding math strategies, see Roditi and Steinberg (2007).

RHYMES

Teachers can help students with the organization and planning stages of this process as specific facts or groups of facts are identified and rhymes are created. Many students learn quickly to create their own rhymes. The Internet is a valuable resource for accessing rhymes for math fact practice. A few examples of rhymes for math facts are listed below:

> 6 and 7 were mighty blue until they met 42.
>
> 6 and 8 met at gate 48.
>
> (from *Math in Bloom: Multiplication/Division*;
> Schroeder & Washington, 1989)

> He stood in line and ate a ton, 9 times 9 is 81.
>
> 6 asked 8 for a date, 6 times 8 is 48.
>
> (from *www.multiplication.com*)

VISUAL REPRESENTATIONS

Visual representations are another way to attach meaning to math facts that are difficult to recall automatically. For some students, pictures can be recalled more easily than verbal descriptions alone. Also, concrete images are easier to remember than abstract concepts. For example, in Figure 5.3, the visual representation of the three M's shows students that when a reference is made to multiples, they are looking for numbers of increasing value. Therefore, Multiples Make More.

Visual representations are often combined with the use of rhymes (or crazy phrases), but they can also be used in isolation (see examples of crazy phrases below). The facts are practiced by repeating the rhymes or crazy phrases and recalling the visuals.

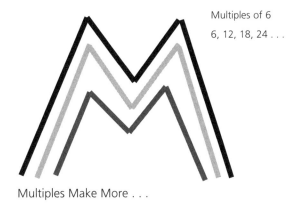

FIGURE 5.3. Multiples Make More strategy.

VISUAL–KINESTHETIC STRATEGIES

Visual–kinesthetic strategies, such as the one pictured below, help students who learn more easily through movement. Even middle and high school students can benefit from this type of active involvement in a lesson.

> *Human number line*: When you hit a plus (+) sign, keep walking the same way. When you hit a minus (–) sign, turn around.

Examples: 4 + 2   –6 + 4   4 + (–2)   –6 –4   5– (–2)

CRAZY PHRASES

Crazy phrases are helpful for remembering operations in a specific order. Many different crazy phrases have been used over the years to teach students the steps in long division: Divide, Multiply, Subtract, and Bring down. Two examples are Dracula's Mother Sucks Blood and Dumb Monkeys Sell Bananas. Similarly, many students (and adults) who have trouble remembering high-value Roman numerals can use the crazy phrase Lucky Cows Drink Milk to remember the symbols and progression of the numerals from smallest to largest.

Lucky	L	= 50
Cows	C	= 100
Drink	D	= 500
Milk	M	= 1,000

Memory Strategies for Math Formulae and Procedures

Many students encounter difficulties in math when they are required to call on their working memory to recall specific formulae and procedures for problem solving. The following strategies are useful for remembering important steps. Students with poor working memory also benefit from recording their strategies in strategy notebooks (see Chapters 2 and 4), which allow them easy access to model problems, examples, and mnemonics that help them to remember the specific steps involved in complex math procedures.

- *Songs* help students to remember rules and recipes, such as the steps for adding and subtracting integers. It is helpful to use melodies that are already familiar to students. Many math websites provide words for familiar songs to help students remember math facts and procedures. The following example uses the melody of

"Row, Row, Row Your Boat" to teach students the steps to solve addition and subtraction problems with integers.

> Same sign, add and keep,
> Different sign, subtract.
> Take the sign of the higher number,
> Then it'll be exact!

- *Stories* can be used to help students memorize formulae such as the conversion from Fahrenheit to Celsius/Centigrade: "Friday (F) is the same as (=) the 9 to 5 (9/5) drag in college (C), and (+) I've only got 32 minutes to go!" ($F = 9/5C + 32$) (Higbee, 1988).
- *Acronyms* such as BEDMAS are used by math students to remind them of the order of operations. BEDMAS stands for Brackets, Exponentials, Division, Multiplication, Addition, Subtraction.
- *FOIL and Face* are common strategies for students to remember how to factor polynomials (see Figure 5.4). FOIL is taught as an acronym for multiplying the First terms, Outside terms, Inside terms, and Last terms. Face is an alternative visual strategy for students who cannot remember the FOIL trick, or who typically make sign errors when they are adding the middle terms (Roditi & Steinberg, 2007).

Memory Strategies for Word Problems

As previously mentioned, problem solving requires students to access, hold, and manipulate multiple pieces of information at one time, which places a major demand on the working memory system. For example, students need to read a

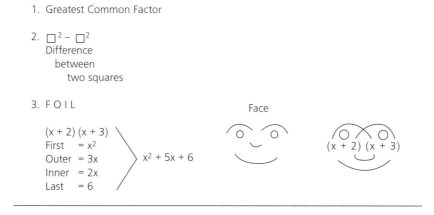

FIGURE 5.4. Factoring strategies.

problem, understand what the problem is asking, decide on the operation(s) to be used, remember facts and procedures, calculate correctly, follow steps, eliminate extraneous information, answer the right question, and finally check their answer. Working memory difficulties can hinder students during any or all of these steps. Weaknesses with automatic memory can also compound the difficulties. The use of paper and pencil to record information as students work through a problem is crucial. Many students with excellent mathematical ability and rote memory often try to avoid writing information down and prefer to solve problems in their heads. As students encounter more complex problems or higher levels of math courses, however, their ability to solve problems efficiently and accurately in this way decreases. Writing down the steps frees up their working memory and increases students' ability to solve problems correctly. In addition to writing down each of the steps, students' ability to solve problems with greater efficiency and accuracy can be achieved by approaching the problems in the following manner. As students encounter a new problem, they should first read the problem carefully and underline key words or directions that are essential to finding the solution. These words may refer to operations to be used, explicitly or implicitly, or may refer to specific problem-solving procedures. Second, students should number the steps in the problem to help them to remember to complete each of them. Last, students should underline the question(s) that are to be answered. The following acronyms can help students to remember key steps and ease the demands for working memory as they solve word problems (Roditi & Steinberg, 2007).

- The CUPS (Circle, Underline, Picture, Solve) strategy is a simple one for elementary students and helps to bring their attention to the key elements of a word problem. Students identify and Circle direction words, Underline (and often number) the steps involved in the problem, Draw a picture, and then Solve.
- The KNOW strategy (Steinberg, 2005) is useful for elementary and middle school students. It focuses their attention on the numbers and operations involved in the problem:

> Key words or phrases
> Numbers that I need
> Operation(s)
> Work it out!
> (See Appendix 9 for a KNOW template.)

- The RAPS (Read and rephrase, Art, Plan and predict, Solve) strategy helps students to break down the components of a word problem and record information in words and pictures. Like the other problem-solving strategies, RAPS allows students with working memory difficulties to improve their ability to work through problems systematically and accurately, and lessens the pressure to remember information mentally. (See Appendix 10 for a RAPS template.)

Memory Strategies for Checking

Self-checking procedures are described in detail in Chapter 7. These strategies are crucial for students who have difficulty knowing and remembering what they should be looking for when they arrive at the checking stage. Not surprisingly, students with executive function weaknesses often skip this stage. Targeted strategies, such as personalized checklists in subject areas, allow students to focus on very specific parts of the assignment when checking for accuracy. In addition, mnemonics or visuals, such as the one described below, can aid recall.

The POUNCE (Pens, Operation, Underline, Number and signs, Calculate, Estimation) strategy (Roditi & Steinberg, 2007) begins with students' physically and mentally making the shift to checking by first changing their pen color (or pen).

Pens	Change pen color for checking
Operation	Did I use the right operation
Underline	Underline the question asked
Numbers and signs	Did I select the right number?
	Did I use the right Sign?
Calculate	Did I calculate correctly?
Estimation	Does my answer agree with an estimate?

Memory Strategies for Studying and Test Taking

Studying for tests is another area that can be overwhelming for many students with memory difficulties. What does "studying" really mean? For many students, studying means reading their notes again and again, in the hope that the information will automatically become lodged in their brains! For this reason, students need to be taught explicitly how to prepare for tests. They need to learn that the steps involved in effective preparation—from daily reading and note taking, to creating mnemonics for remembering vocabulary or math procedures, to using checking procedures consistently—are all part of the studying–learning continuum. The strategies summarized in Table 5.4 and described below can be used to teach students how to study and take tests effectively.

Organizing and Remembering Strategies for Studying

CHUNKING TOGETHER RELATED INFORMATION

Chunking together is a useful strategy for organizing and recalling essential information. For instance, in history, students can identify names, places, and events that go together. Subsequently, these chunks of information can be linked in a verbal (story form) or visual (graphic) manner, depending on students' learning

TABLE 5.4. Memory Strategies for Studying and Test Taking

Focus area	Strategy	Purpose
Studying	Chunking Strategy cards	To create and record various strategies for remembering

	Memory joggers
	  Crazy phrases
	  Silly sentences
	  Acronyms
	Stories
	Rhymes and songs
	Triple Note Tote
		To recall difficult information

Test taking	Brain Dump	To lessen working memory demands
	QUEST	To check essay answers for completeness

Note. See text for explanation of QUEST.

style. See Figure 5.5 for a student's graphic representation of major ideas related to the study of abolitionism.

STRATEGY CARDS

Strategy cards go beyond the commonly used index card or flash card format. Their purpose is to have students identify both the content information they are required to know and a strategy for recalling that piece of information. See Fig-

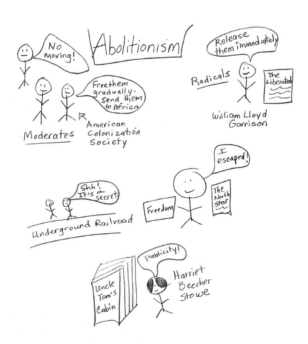

FIGURE 5.5. Graphic representation of abolitionism.

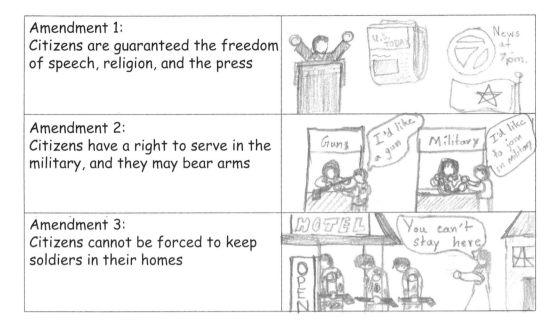

Amendment 1: Citizens are guaranteed the freedom of speech, religion, and the press	
Amendment 2: Citizens have a right to serve in the military, and they may bear arms	
Amendment 3: Citizens cannot be forced to keep soldiers in their homes	

FIGURE 5.6. Example of a strategy card for the Bill of Rights: Amendments (at left) on the front, pictures to aid in recall (at right) on the back.

ure 5.6 for an example created by a high school student to remember the first 10 Amendments to the U.S. Constitution (the Bill of Rights). On the front of each card, some of the amendments were stated. On the reverse side, the student drew pictures that would help him to recall the specific details of the amendments.

OTHER "MEMORY JOGGERS"

Strategies such as crazy phrases, silly sentences, and acronyms, are useful when students are required to memorize long lists of items or a process. The sillier or more absurd the mnemonic, the greater the chance of recalling that information. The addition of a visual representation, such as a cartoon or diagram, is useful for many students. When any of these memory joggers are being used, frequent practice and rehearsal are important to facilitate recall. Examples of content-related memory joggers are listed in Table 5.5.

STORIES

Stories are also useful strategies for remembering a large number of items or information at one time. In order to recall the 13 original colonies, the following story can be used.

There's a cow named Georgia (Georgia)

It's a Jersey cow (New Jersey)

She's singing a couple of Christmas carols
(North and South Carolina)

Under her arm is a Virginia ham (Virginia,
New Hampshire)

The cow is wearing a pair of yellow underwear
(Delaware)

In its hoof is a pencil (Pennsylvania)

The cow is making a connect-the-dots picture
(Connecticut)

Of Marilyn Monroe (Maryland)

Walking down the road (Rhode Island)

Going to Mass (Massachusetts)

TABLE 5.5. Types of Memory Joggers and Functions

Strategy	Purpose/examples	Content information
Crazy phrase	A made-up wacky phrase to help remember names, places, or events in a specific order	
	<u>M</u>innie and <u>I</u> were <u>M</u>iserable <u>W</u>earing <u>I</u>tchy <u>M</u>ittens <u>I</u>nside <u>O</u>ut	To recall the eight Midwest states: Minnesota, Iowa, Missouri, Wisconsin, Illinois, Michigan, Indiana, Ohio
Silly sentence	A nonsensical sentence to help remember key names or concepts	
	<u>B</u>rave <u>S</u>ailors <u>G</u>ot <u>V</u>ery <u>C</u>old <u>E</u>ggs (BrainCogs)	To recall the names and locations of countries in the northern part of South America: Brazil, Suriname, Guyana, Venezuela, Columbia, Ecuador
	That crazy <u>weatherman</u> said the temperature would <u>cool</u> down, but the <u>heat</u> was so intense that we could <u>melt</u> a candy bar on the <u>cement</u> (Gibson, 2006).	To remember the five processes in the rock cycle: weathering, cooling, heat, melting, cementation
Acronym	A real or nonsense word (or words) in which each letter stands for the first letter of a key word; sometimes a letter is inserted in order to make a word	
	ANN E. BOA (BrainCogs)	To help remember seven tricky words to be aware of on tests: <u>A</u>lways, <u>N</u>ever, <u>N</u>ot, <u>E</u>xcept, <u>B</u>ut, <u>O</u>nly, and <u>A</u>ll
	RED CRaNES (BrainCogs)	To help remember the systems of the human body: <u>R</u>eproductive, <u>E</u>xcretory, <u>D</u>igestive, <u>C</u>irculatory, <u>R</u>espiratory, <u>N</u>ervous, <u>E</u>ndocrine, and <u>S</u>keletal

RHYMES AND SONGS

As previously noted in the discussion of memory strategies for math, the use of rhymes and songs can improve memory for factual information across academic domains and for students at all grade levels. In social studies, for example, a student can make up a rhyme to remember specific events and dates (e.g., "In 1765, the Stamp Act was alive").

TRIPLE NOTE TOTE

Triple Note Tote from BrainCogs (ResearchILD & FableVision, 2003), previously described in Chapter 2, is also an effective study tool. After the content information is organized, students can add a memory jogger in the third column for the items that they have the most difficulty remembering. For some content information, a memory aid is not needed, because the student is able to recall the information easily. See the Triple Note Tote example in Figure 5.7 for use of memory joggers related to a science unit.

Again, with each of these strategies, students need to repeatedly practice and rehearse both, orally and in writing, in order to maximize their chances for effective and efficient recall.

Memory Strategies for Test Taking

BRAIN DUMP

When handed a test, students can immediately write down memory joggers and other information that they are likely to forget, such as math formulae or challeng-

Main tissue types	Example and description	Memory jogger
Epithelial	Skin Covers outside of body, lines inner surfaces of body	Sounds like "upper-sealing," skin seals your body
Connective	Ligaments, cartilage, blood Fills in spaces, connects things, supports and insulates organs	The name (connective) tells what it does. To remember the examples, a "CLuB" connects people: C = cartilage, L = ligaments, B = blood

FIGURE 5.7. Example of the use memory joggers in Triple Note Tote.

ing vocabulary definitions. Recording this information at the tops of their papers lessens the demands on their working memory and often decreases their level of anxiety.

QUEST TO DO YOUR BEST!

The QUEST strategy helps students to remember where they should direct their attention when they finish their work.

QU—Read the Question carefully:
  • Did you answer all parts of the question?
E—Look at your Evidence:
  • Did I include at least three details, such as examples, dates, vocabulary words, names, arguments?
S—Check for Signal words:
  • Did I use signal words to clarify order and transitions, such as "However," "The main reason," "Finally"?
T—Look over your Topic sentences:
  • Does each paragraph have a good topic sentence?
  • Did I start my essay with a topic sentence that introduces the main idea?

Accommodations for Working Memory Deficits

Strategies are not always sufficient for ensuring students' success in school. Weaknesses in one or more areas, such as working memory, attention, processing speed, and visual–motor skills, make many tasks challenging for students. Working memory, in particular, has a significant impact on academic performance, and students with weaknesses in this area often find it challenging to retain and manipulate needed information while simultaneously producing work (e.g., writing, taking notes, answering test questions). Some students may require specific accommodations in conjunction with strategy instruction to enable them to access the curriculum and meet the demands of their classes. Examples of *general* accommodations for students with working memory weaknesses include the following:

  • A designated class note taker
  • Recording of lectures
  • Access to the instructor's PowerPoint presentations
  • Word banks
  • Visual checklists and "to-do" lists on Post-it Notes
  • Graphic organizers for writing

Examples of *subject-specific* accommodations include the following:

- *Math*: Calculator, procedure lists, multiplication chart
- *Reading*: Recorded books, electronic readers
- *Written expression*: Word processor, electronic writing organizers or templates, grammar and spell-check tools, writing rubrics

CONCLUSION

The ability to retain, retrieve, and mentally manipulate information is essential for learning. Students with executive function difficulties may exhibit weaknesses in memory, particularly in working memory, that compromise their ability to learn and remember information and to perform at the level of their potential. Thus effective strategy instruction tailored to diverse learning profiles is critically important for maximizing students' learning. The use of research-based memory strategies, such as chunking, crazy phrases, acronyms, cartoons, songs, rhymes, and stories, provides students with the tools to overcome their working memory weaknesses and increase their academic success. In turn, students' success requires educators to be thoughtful in their selection of critical information and the strategies students need to remember content information and procedures. As a result of careful planning and systematic strategy instruction, students can learn to "work smarter" and more efficiently.

CHAPTER 6

Shifting and Flexible Problem Solving

The Anchors for Academic Success

LYNN MELTZER and JENNIFER SAGE BAGNATO

Middle school has been especially challenging for Leo. When he's doing his homework, he seems to understand the concepts and information presented in his science textbook. However, he can't seem to apply this information on tests and extend it to new scenarios. I try to help him in math, but he gets frustrated when I show him an approach that is different from the way he was taught in school. He gets stuck doing things over and over again the same way, so that homework drags on the entire night, and he gets too little sleep. Even after he works so hard, his grades are still lower than those of his friends, and Leo now tells us that his friends are much smarter than he is.

—PARENT OF A SIXTH GRADER

Sally's performance in school is like a seesaw. She is a very hard worker and is diligent with her homework. When taking notes, she spends hours writing down every detail. However, she sometimes has difficulty with broad concepts and struggles to find the main ideas in her English literature and social studies assignments. When writing essays, she frequently includes quotes and specific examples that don't relate to her thesis. Sally does well on multiple-choice tests and fill-in-the-blank quizzes. I do not understand why she has so much difficulty with short-answer and essay tests, and I wish I knew how to help Sally so that her grades were more representative of the time and effort she spends studying.

—11TH-GRADE TEACHER

*C*ognitive flexibility, or the ability to think without rigidity and to shift mindsets easily, is a critically important executive function process that is often especially challenging for students like Sally, Leo, and others with learning and attention difficulties (Meltzer, 1993; Meltzer & Krishnan, 2007; Meltzer & Montague, 2001; Meltzer, Solomon, Fenton, & Levine, 1989). Its component processes—which include the ability to adapt to unfamiliar or unexpected situations, to combine concepts creatively, and to integrate different representations—develop across the lifespan and vary among students (Cartwright, 2008a, 2008b, 2008c; Deák, 2008). Many academic tasks from early elementary school into high school require students to shift flexibly between perspectives and to synthesize information in novel ways (see Chapters 1 and 2). Nevertheless, time is usually not built into the curriculum for teaching students the importance of approaching problem solving and academic tasks flexibly, so they can shift easily "from the top of the mountain to the bottom" as they focus alternately on the major themes and the relevant details (see Figure 1.1 in Chapter 1).

In this chapter, we discuss the reasons *why* cognitive flexibility is so important across the grades, and in all academic domains. We also provide an overview of specific strategies that teachers can implement in their classrooms to help students approach complex problems in a flexible manner, integrate multiple representations of knowledge, and apply learned skills to novel situations. Some of the suggestions discussed in this chapter, like some of those in other chapters, have been evaluated as part of our school-based *Gateways to Success* and *Drive to Thrive* studies (Meltzer et al., 2004a, 2004b, 2004c). Others are based on considerable clinical research (Meltzer et al., 2007b) or on best practice. Teachers could use these strategies as guides in devising their own approaches for helping students to develop flexible mindsets in the different content areas.

WHY IS COGNITIVE FLEXIBILITY SO IMPORTANT ACROSS GRADES AND ACADEMIC DOMAINS?

Children's ability to think flexibly changes with development and age (Brown, 1997; Cartwright, 2008a, 2008b). Typically, students in the early elementary grades have a more limited understanding of the importance of using different approaches to their work in different situations than do middle and high school students. In fact, recent research has shown that cognitive-developmental changes from childhood into adulthood influence children's ability to manage the cognitive complexity of academic tasks and to process many different elements simultaneously (Andrews & Halford, 2002; Cartwright, 2008a, 2008b; Zelazo & Müller, 2002).

As children enter school, cognitive flexibility plays an increasingly important role in the development of more advanced language and literacy skills (Cartwright, 2002, 2008a, 2008b; Homer & Hayward, 2008). Furthermore, the acquisition of numeracy skills is increasingly linked with students' ability to process multiple representations flexibly and easily. Acquisition of new concepts is also connected to students' willingness to abandon previously successful approaches in favor of alternative methods when necessary (Cartwright, 2008a, 2008b). This ability to shift approaches and to synthesize information in novel ways is essential for effective reading, writing, math problem solving, note taking, studying, and test taking.

In the reading domain, investigators have recently emphasized the importance of *reading flexibility*, or readers' ability to adapt their reading skills to the demands and purpose of the material (Adams, 1990; Fry, 1978; Cartwright, 2002; Gaskins, 2008; Wagner & Sternberg, 1987). This emphasis on the role of cognitive flexibility in reading decoding, fluency, and comprehension reflects the multidimensional nature of reading (Berninger, Abbott, Thomson, & Raskind, 2001; Berninger & Nagy, 2008; Gaskins, 2008, Gaskins, Satlow, & Pressley, 2007; Pressley, 2006). As reading tasks become more challenging and domain-specific, students need to coordinate multiple subskills, processes, and sources of information. They form mental representations that they need to access flexibly in order to remember, organize, prioritize, and comprehend the information (Shanahan & Shanahan, 2008).

Accurate and efficient reading decoding requires students to shift flexibly among four different approaches: letter–sound decoding, use of sight word vocabulary, reliance on context clues, and use of analogies (Ehri, 1991; Gaskins, 2008). In other words, they need to recognize the importance of what Gaskins (2008) refers to as "crisscrossing the landscape," in order to select decoding approaches that fit the text. Specifically, students need to coordinate the letter–sound relationships with the meanings of printed words (Cartwright, 2002, 2008a, 2008b, 2008c). When studies have focused on teaching students to shift flexibly as part of the decoding process, findings have shown improved reading decoding and comprehension in beginning readers, intermediate readers, and adults (Cartwright, 2002, 2008a, 2008b, 2008c). Other studies have shown the efficacy of teaching students different approaches to decoding and fostering flexibility in decoding (Lovett, Lacerenza, & Borden, 2000). Such flexibility helps students coordinate and shift between word-level features on the one hand, and vocabulary knowledge and background knowledge on the other. This flexibility allows students to draw inferences that extend beyond the information given, and thus it facilitates reading comprehension (Adams, 1990; Cartwright, 2008a, 2008b, 2008c).

Reading comprehension requires students to process the meaning of text, flexibly access their background knowledge, recognize the purpose or goal of reading (Cartwright, 2008a, 2008b, 2008c), and monitor their own comprehension (Block & Pressley, 2002; Pressley & Afflerbach, 1995). Reading for meaning taxes students' ability to manage linguistic information at the word, sentence, and paragraph levels (Brown & Deavers, 1999; Goswami, Ziegler, Dalton, & Schneider, 2001, 2003). In the well-known series of books about Amelia Bedelia, for example, young readers need to use a flexible approach to language in order to understand the multiple meanings of the language embedded in the text and the humor in the stories. This flexibility helps readers to understand why Amelia Bedelia's employers are surprised when they come home to find a chicken dressed in clothes after they ask her to "Dress the chicken," and a drawing of their curtains and light bulbs on the front lawn after they ask her to "Draw the drapes when the sun comes in . . . and put the lights out" (Parish, 1963, pp. 47, 48, 59).

Written language, like reading comprehension, requires students to shift—in this case, between the topic sentences on the one hand, and the supporting details on the other. As students learn to shift approaches flexibly, they are able to interpret information in more than one way, change approaches when needed, and choose a new strategy when the first one is not working (Westman & Kamoo, 1990). There is still a need for longitudinal studies that focus on the impact of cognitive flexibility on the writing process, as there has been very little research in this area.

In the math domain, students' understanding of concepts, of computational procedures, and of word problems is associated with cognitive flexibility from the earliest grades, when one-to-one correspondence rules are taught. Students need to shift from the words and sentences in math problems to the numbers, operations, algorithms, and equations needed to solve the problems (Roditi & Steinberg, 2007). Students also need to learn how and when to shift from one problem-solving strategy or schema to another, so that their final calculations are accurate and logical (Montague & Jitendra, 2006). In fact, recent math curricula that have been based on the National Council of Teachers of Math (2000) report focus on teaching students to switch sets while they connect, communicate, and discuss multiple representations of the same word problems. Students with learning disabilities often struggle to shift flexibly between the numbers and the math questions they are solving (Bull & Scerif, 2001; Roditi, 1993; Roditi & Steinberg, 2007). Therefore, these students need explicit and ongoing instruction in shifting when they approach their math work.

In content area subjects, including science and history, students are required to read texts where many words or phrases have multiple meanings; students' understanding of these words or phrases depends on their flexible use of context clues. Similarly, learning a foreign language requires a significant amount of flexible thinking, as students are challenged to shift back and forth between their native language and the language they are learning. Students continuously need to apply their knowledge of semantics, syntax, and vocabulary in order to translate text or conversation in the foreign language into their native language and vice versa. Spiro and colleagues have stressed the role of flexibility in the acquisition and representation of content area knowledge (Spiro, 2004; Spiro, Feltovich, Jacobson, & Coulson, 1992). Specifically, they have shown that knowledge needs to be flexibly structured and accessed in order to build expertise in different academic domains. Cognitive flexibility and other higher-level thinking skills therefore need to be explicitly taught within specific content domains or disciplines (Shanahan & Shanahan, 2008). In fact, in studies of the links between cognitive flexibility and performance in science and history, students across the grades (elementary into high school) have been taught to shift flexibly among texts and to recognize similarities and differences in themes, in order to understand the main ideas or "big picture" (Shanahan & Shanahan, 2008; Wolfe & Goldman, 2005).

Finally, note taking, studying, and taking tests require students to shift back and forth between various subtopics or problem types, which are often phrased differently from the ways in which students have learned or studied the information. In these different academic domains, students with learning difficulties need to learn systematic strategies for interpreting the vocabulary and linguistic structure in multiple ways, so that they feel comfortable taking risks and thinking "outside the box" when they interpret information.

Across all these academic domains, students' motivation, interest, and passion influence their willingness to make the effort to try different approaches and to shift flexibly from one approach to another, rather than continuing to use the same approach to tasks (Alexander, 1998; Paris, Lipson, & Wixson, 1983; Shanahan & Shanahan, 2008). Alexander (1998) emphasizes that intrinsic motivation, topic knowledge, and strategy use interact to produce improvements in domain learning (e.g., history or science). For example, as students learn more about a topic (such as the Vietnam War), they find it easier to use strategies flexibly; in turn, flexible strategy use increases students' interest in completing the many different steps involved in writing a paper about the Vietnam War. In this regard, Zelazo and colleagues have differentiated between purely cognitive or "cold" tasks that have no emotional content (e.g., math computation) and tasks that are affected by a student's social and emotional mindset, or what they term "hot" tasks (e.g., remembering information in a social studies text by linking it with a personal experience) (Zelazo & Müller, 2002; Zelazo, Müller, Frye, & Marcovitch, 2003). They propose that success on both types of tasks depends on each individual's cognitive flexibility.

HOW SHOULD WE TEACH STUDENTS TO THINK FLEXIBLY AND TO SHIFT MINDSETS?

As discussed above, classroom instruction needs to include opportunities for students to use their acquired knowledge flexibly (Bereiter & Scardamalia, 1993). Similarly, students' cognitive flexibility improves when they are given opportunities to solve problems from a variety of different perspectives (Bransford, Brown, & Cocking, 2000). Therefore, it is important to embed strategies for teaching cognitive flexibility into different facets of the curriculum, and to create classrooms and school cultures where students are taught strategies that encourage flexible thinking across the grades and content areas.

In the classroom setting, cognitive flexibility underlies good teaching as well as successful learning (Cartwright, 2008a, 2008b, 2008c; Massey, 2008). As Massey (2008) emphasizes, "flexible instruction does not mean anything goes" (p. 305). Instead, such instruction provides explicit models of a repertoire of specific strategies, as well as explanations of how and when to use these strategies (Snow, Griffin, & Burns, 2005).

A broad range of instructional methods can be used to promote flexible thinking across the content areas. Instruction can focus explicitly on problem solving and critical thinking, and can require students to think flexibly about how the solutions they propose could lead to different outcomes under different circumstances (Sternberg, 2005). Instruction can also encourage peer discussion and collaborative learning in order to expose students to many different viewpoints (Yuill, 2007; Yuill & Bradwell, 1998). While working with their peers, students can be challenged to approach problems from the perspectives of their classmates, which may vary significantly from their own. An integrated approach to learning encourages students to make connections between different content areas and also challenges them to think flexibly about the topics. For example, in history, when students are taught about the westward migration in the United States during the 1850s, each student could be required to write a journal from the perspective of a pioneer. In geography or science, students could analyze the topographical features of the area and choose a safe passage through the Sierra Nevada. This integrated approach not only deepens students' understanding of the time period, but also encourages them to shift mindsets by assuming a number of different perspectives.

The following guide can be used as an organizational framework for embedding shifting strategies in the curriculum (see Chapter 2 for details):

1. Introduce and define the concept of shifting strategies.
2. Model shifting strategies and explain what, when, and how to do this.
3. Provide opportunities for active student learning.
4. Reinforce shifting strategies by embedding opportunities for doing this into the curriculum.
5. Reflect on students' use of specific strategies.
6. Challenge students and extend flexible strategy use to other academic areas and tasks.

To help students develop metacognitive awareness and understand how to shift flexibly in their interpretation of language and approaches to reading, writing, and math, one of the easiest and most enjoyable activities is to implement "5-minute warm-ups" at the beginning of lessons. These activities encourage students to recognize that many different answers can often be generated for the same question (see Table 6.1 for examples). Furthermore, activities with jokes, riddles, word categories, and number puzzles can help students to practice using flexible approaches to language interpretation and number manipulation.

Tasks that incorporate jokes and riddles "differentiate between what is said and what is meant, between two different meanings of the same surface form, between joking and literal interpretations of text, and between formal and semantic characteristics of words" (Yuill, Kerawalla, Pearce, Luckin, & Harris, 2008, p. 339). The efficacy of using jokes to teach flexible thinking to students in the early grades has

TABLE 6.1. Warm-Up Activities That Promote Flexible Interpretation of Language and Flexible Approaches to Reading, Writing, and Math

- Present ambiguous words and sentences to students in the form of riddles or jokes. This is an enjoyable way of helping students to use context clues to analyze words with multiple meanings. This activity should be linked directly and explicitly with reading comprehension tasks.

- Encourage students to identify different ways they can use specific objects such as a brick, a cardboard box, or an apple. This encourages them to shift approaches rather than getting "stuck" in one approach, and helps them to understand that objects as well as words can have different meanings and functions.

- Ask students to categorize weekly vocabulary or spelling words in a number of different ways (e.g., by part of speech, meaning, vowel patterns).

- Ask students to identify several different ways in which selected multimeaning words can be used (e.g., "*cut* paper" "*cut* the line," "*cut* class."

- Encourage students to write a short story from the perspective of an object, such as a penny or a lost sock. This teaches perspective taking and helps students to shift approaches.

- Ask students to create different endings for books they have read. This process encourages students to recognize that stories can end in many different ways.

- Play word and math logic games, such as Boggle, Magic Squares, and Sudoku, to help students to manipulate words and numbers in different ways and to think flexibly about words and math operations.

been shown in an interesting series of studies (Yuill, 2007; Yuill & Bradwell, 1998). Children ages 7–9 years were paired with peers to discuss ambiguities in jokes; they used a joke software program (Joke City) for three 30-hour sessions. Significant gains in reading comprehension were found in these children, in comparison with the control group children, who continued with their daily literacy classes. In other words, an explicit focus on the ambiguous language in jokes generalized to reading comprehension as students were required to think about and analyze language in different ways.

Jokes and riddles help students to recognize that ambiguities in language affect meaning, and that looking for context clues is an important reading strategy that improves reading comprehension (see Figure 6.1). Ambiguous sentences, riddles, and multimeaning words can be presented in humorous ways to teach students how to shift flexibly among meanings by using context clues, shifting from noun to verb use, and shifting syllables in words. As Yuill et al. (1998) point out, peer

---

Think about and illustrate two different meanings for the following:

- Eye drops off the shelf.
- Enraged cow injures farmer with axe.
- Kids make nutritious snacks.
- Hospitals are sued by seven foot doctors.
- Include your friends when baking cookies.

FIGURE 6.1. Examples of using humor to promote flexible interpretation of multimeaning words.

discussion of jokes promotes cognitive flexibility, as joking is a social activity that occurs among peers. Similarly, peer discussions of ambiguous language promotes metacognitive awareness that transfers to reading and writing tasks (Yuill et al., 2008). Students can therefore collaborate with peers to illustrate or verbally explain selected riddles or jokes. They can also work with peers to analyze sentence structure and to identify pronouns, adjectives, and placements of commas or hyphens that change the meanings of words and phrases. Discussing these different meanings often helps students to recognize the importance of thinking flexibly when they complete their homework or study for tests.

Activities like these provide opportunities to incorporate cognitive flexibility instruction into classwork and homework through the use of enjoyable and inherently motivating tasks. These activities should be linked explicitly and directly with reading comprehension tasks. Therefore, teachers can present reading tasks that require students to recognize shifts in sentence meanings based on the use of selected words as nouns or verbs. Students can be required to discuss these shifts explicitly. In this way, students can use engaging material to build their metacognitive and metalinguistic awareness.

It is important to recognize that students often show marked variability in their cognitive flexibility, and that students may be flexible on some tasks but not on others. For instance, some students may be flexible in their approach to structured verbal or nonverbal reasoning tasks, yet may be inflexible in academic situations that demand the integrated use of a broad range of skills and strategies. Similarly, students may actively use learning strategies on tasks with which they are familiar, but may not access strategies on other tasks that they perceive as too difficult or that require the simultaneous mobilization of multiple processes and strategies. They may also rely inappropriately on strategies that were previously helpful, but are inadequate for dealing with the increased complexity of new tasks. Teachers can differentiate instruction more easily after administering the Meta-COG surveys (see Chapter 1 for a detailed discussion of MetaCOG) to assess all students' motivation, effort, strategy use, and understanding of their own learning profiles. Students' motivation and emotional mindsets (e.g., fatigue, anxiety, social awareness) influence their willingness to make the extra effort needed to use strategies for thinking and learning flexibly. In fact, as discussed in detail in Chapter 8, students' emotional mindsets often serve as "on–off switches" for effective strategy use and learning, particularly their willingness to try new or different approaches.

Table 6.2 provides suggestions for teaching students to develop metacognitive mindsets—to shift flexibly "from the top of the mountain to the bottom and back again" (see Chapter 1), and to shift between the main ideas and details in different content areas and domains. These broad ideas are expanded and elaborated in the following section, which focuses on *what* strategies teachers should use to promote students' abilities to think flexibly and to shift approaches as needed.

TABLE 6.2. Teaching Students to Develop Metacognitive Mindsets and Strategies for Shifting Flexibly in Selected Content Areas

Oral language

Shifting between multiple word meanings

- Teach students to recognize and analyze ambiguities in words and sentences, and to shift between different meanings.
- Require students to identify multiple-meaning words by using context clues, noun–verb clues, and syllable accents, and to shift flexibly among the different possible meanings (see the M & M strategy, Figures 6/4–6.5 and Table 6.3).
- Explicitly link these activities with reading comprehension and writing, so that students will generalize and extend the strategies they learn to the different content areas.

Reading decoding and spelling

Shifting between different word analysis and blending approaches for decoding and spelling

- Teach students to recognize which words can be analyzed by using phonics and which words depend on sight vocabulary.
- Provide sentence-reading tasks where students need to shift between phonics and sight words. Require students to verbalize the difference, so that they develop a metacognitive approach to decoding and spelling.
- Teach students to access their knowledge of prefixes and suffixes and related words in spelling—for example, *music*/*musical* (*c* at the end, not *k* or *ck*); *jumped* (*ed*, not *t*, because of past tense).

Note: Students sometimes rely exclusively on phonics if they are not taught how and when to shift strategies.

Reading comprehension

Shifting between "big ideas" and supporting details

- Teach students to differentiate among main ideas, important details, and less relevant details. This is an important skill for summarizing and studying.
- Require students to identify multiple-meaning words, as above.
- Teach students to use three-column notes (e.g., Triple Note Tote), to ensure that they shift from the main ideas or core concepts to the supportive details (see Chapter 2).

Written language

Shifting between "big ideas" and supporting details.

Shifting "from the top to the bottom of the mountain and back again" (see Chapters 1 and 2)

- Provide students with graphic organizers for sorting main ideas vs. supportive details.
- Provide templates that help students focus on major themes or thesis statements, relevant details, and conclusions.
- Provide models for shifting from the main ideas to supporting details.
- Help students to develop personalized checklists that help them differentiate between relevant and irrelevant details.

Studying and test taking

Shifting and organizing

Shifting and self-checking

- Have students create specific study plans for tests in different subject areas and with different formats (e.g., essay vs. multiple-choice).
- Have students use a question–answer or three-column format (e.g., Triple Note Tote) for studying for tests.
- Have students shift from writing to editing, using personalized checklists of their common errors on tests.

(cont.)

TABLE 6.2. *(cont.)*

<u>Summarizing, note taking, long-term projects</u>

Shifting and prioritizing

Shifting and organizing

- Teach the "big picture" versus the details by using concept maps and reminding students to visualize themselves standing at the "top of the mountain" and then shifting to the "bottom of the mountain" for the details.
- Teach students to extract the main themes when taking notes and to paraphrase the information in their own words.
- Require students to use the Triple Note Tote strategy or strategy cards throughout each chapter/unit (see Chapter 2). These require students to shift from the main ideas to the details and back again, so that they have a study plan for tests.
- Require students to shift between short-term homework due immediately and long-term projects by using monthly and weekly calendars and setting short-term "due dates" for phases of the long-term work.

<u>Math Problem Solving</u>

Shifting and prioritizing

- Require students to generate math language for each operation (e.g., *difference, less, take away* = subtraction).
- Teach students to shift from the language embedded in word problems to the computational details and back again.
- Teach students to focus on the meaning of the math problem versus the operations and calculation details by reminding students to visualize themselves standing at the "top of the mountain" and then shifting to the "bottom of the mountain" for the details.
- Within operations (e.g., long division) teach students to shift from division to subtraction (and the like).
- Require students to estimate the answers to word problems ("big picture") and to compare their solutions with their estimates. Teach students to ask themselves, " Does it make sense?", by comparing their final calculations with their estimates.

WHAT STRATEGIES SHOULD WE TEACH TO PROMOTE STUDENTS' COGNITIVE FLEXIBILITY?

Specific strategies for fostering flexible thinking and set shifting are often embedded in classroom instruction, but may not be explicitly taught. Students are often unaware of the goals of the lessons or activities, and metacognitive awareness is not actively promoted. The following suggestions and strategies should be used as guides for *explicitly* helping students to develop flexible mindsets and approaches to the different content areas.

Shifting and Flexible Thinking in Reading

As discussed above, reading tasks require students to apply and combine different strategies on the basis of the specific goals, text structures, and content requirements of the different tasks (Brown et al., 1983). When reading novels, for example, students are required to shift between the concrete and the abstract, between the literal and the symbolic, and between the major themes and relevant details. Similarly, students regularly encounter ambiguous language when they read poetry, and texts in content areas such as biology or history which also require them to think flexibly about the meanings of specific words, phrases, and sentences. There are three major categories of ambiguous language (Spector, 1997):

- *Multiple-meaning words.* These include homographs and homophones, such as *pair* versus *pear* and *weight* versus *wait*. Changing the accent of a word may also vary the meaning of words, as in the example of *PROduce* versus *proDUCE*.
- *Multiple-meaning phrases.* Ambiguous phrases are often idioms, such as "eats like a bird," "break a leg," "follow your heart", and "off the wall."
- *Multiple-meaning sentences.* To interpret ambiguous sentences, readers must use syntactic information and context clues embedded in the text to infer the correct meaning. For oral language, listeners may also analyze verbal cues (e.g., stress and intonation) and nonverbal cues (e.g., gestures and body language) to understand the intended meanings of the sentences. They also need to identify which specific parts of sentences can be interpreted in two different ways. Examples include "Jane has grown another foot" and "He grimaced when Ralph took his picture."

Students need to learn how to recognize and analyze multimeaning words, phrases, and sentences, and how to use context clues to shift back and forth between the main ideas and the details.

As discussed above, many approaches can be used. For example, riddles, multimeaning words, and ambiguous sentences can be presented in humorous ways to teach students how to shift flexibly among meanings by using context clues, shifting from noun to verb use, or shifting accents or syllables in words. Teachers can present students with jokes or riddles such as those shown in Figures 6.2 and 6.3, and can require students to do the following:

- Read the jokes or riddles.
- Identify the literal and figurative meanings of the words.
- Underline the part of the joke with multiple meanings.

- What did the ocean say to the shore?
  Nothing, it just waved.

- What did the calculator say to the student?
  You can count on me.

- What do you get when you eat crackers in bed?
  A crumby night's sleep.

- Why shouldn't you step on a watch?
  Because it's a waste of time.

FIGURE 6.2. Examples of using riddles to promote flexible interpretation of multimeaning words.

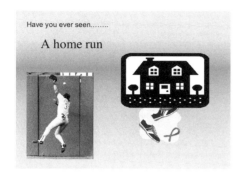
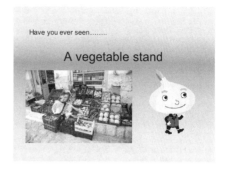

FIGURE 6.3. Teaching cognitive flexibility by illustrating words or phrases in which multiple meanings are associated with verb or noun usage.

- Illustrate the two or more different meanings by hand or on a computer.
- Discuss the multiple meanings with peer partners.

Strategies like the *multiple-meaning strategy* (M & M strategy) can also help students to unlock the meaning of ambiguous language. To use the M & M strategy, students are encouraged to follow the steps outlined in Figure 6.4.

As discussed in detail in Chapter 5, students need memory anchors to remember sequences of steps. Crazy phrases that link the steps in a sequence can often help students to recall the order in which they need to analyze the material. For example, to remember the steps involved in the M & M strategy, students could be presented with one of the following crazy phrases: "Mighty Pandas Crave Large Oreos" (see Figure 6.5), "Mean Possums Crush Lollipops Ominously," or "Mischie-

---

Multiple-meaning word—Check each *unfamiliar* or confusing word in the sentence and ask:

- Could this word have more than one meaning?
- Could it be used as both a verb and a noun?
- Can I change the accent or stress of the word?

Possible meanings—List all the possible meanings of the word.

Context clues—Circle and analyze context clues in the sentences.

Logical meaning—Underline the most logical meaning. Cross out meanings that don't make sense.

Own words: Restate the sentence in your own words.

Crazy phrase: "Mighty Pandas Crave Large Oreos."

FIGURE 6.4. The multiple-meaning strategy (M & M strategy).

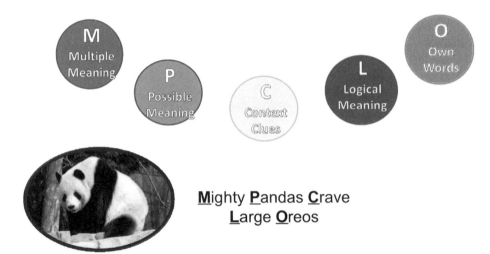

Mighty Pandas Crave Large Oreos

FIGURE 6.5. Use of a crazy phrase to recall the M & M Strategy for shifting flexibly among multiple word meanings.

vous Penguins Collect Lopsided Oranges." Once they have practiced using the M& M strategy, students should be encouraged to make up their own crazy phrases. Table 6.3 demonstrates how students might use the M & M strategy to comprehend the following ambiguous sentence: "The hiker looked at the scale carefully."

While ambiguous language challenges students to think flexibly at the word and sentence levels, students are also required to shift mindsets when reading paragraphs in textbooks and chapters in novels. To comprehend fiction, for example, it is important that readers shift mindsets to think like the characters in a book. Consider the following excerpt from page 1 of *The Ballad of Lucy Whipple*, by Karen Cushman (1996):

> It was a hot day in late August, and nothing was moving in the heat but the flies, when our wagon pulled out of the woods and stopped at the edge of the ravine.

TABLE 6.3. Using the M & M Strategy to Comprehend Ambiguous Language

Ambiguity	Possible meanings	Context clues	Logical meaning	Own words
The hiker looked at the scale carefully.	• Machine for weighing • Plate on fish or reptiles • Proportion on a map • To climb up • Series of musical tones	• *hiker*—suggests that the scale is something one might need in the wilderness • *the*—suggests that scale is a noun • *carefully*—suggests that the scale is important to the hiker; it might be hard to see	• Machine for weighing • Plate on fish or reptiles • Proportion on a map • To climb up • Series of musical tones	• The hiker looked at the proportion on the map carefully.

When this passage is interpreted from a contemporary perspective, readers might assume that "our wagon" refers to a station wagon (i.e., a car). However, if the readers are able to shift mindsets and leave behind the time and place in which they live in favor of those in the book (California in 1848), it is more likely that they will activate their background knowledge about this time period and visualize a wooden, horse-drawn wagon. Similarly, in order for readers to understand and analyze a character's actions, they must discard their personal goals/values and temporarily adopt those of the main character. Use of a Venn diagram helps students to make this shift. This approach makes explicit the differences between the readers and the main character, and students need to think about the similarities and differences when they draw the Venn. To help readers change mindsets, students can be encouraged to refer to the Venn diagram before each reading session. Figure 6.6 is an example of a structured and scaffolded Venn diagram that focuses on the setting.

Shifting and Flexible Thinking in Written Language

Persuasive and analytical writing requires students to develop an argument or thesis, which is supported by specific evidence and examples. To facilitate planning and organization, writers are often required to complete a linear graphic organizer that outlines their main idea and supporting details. For some students, this is an effective approach. However, for those who have difficulty with flexible thinking, it may be challenging for them to shift fluidly between their main ideas and supporting details. Consequently, they may choose examples (such as quotes or facts) that either lend little support to the main idea or are entirely unrelated. Use of a graphic organizer that makes explicit connections between the main idea and supporting details may help writers to shift more fluidly between the two (see Appen-

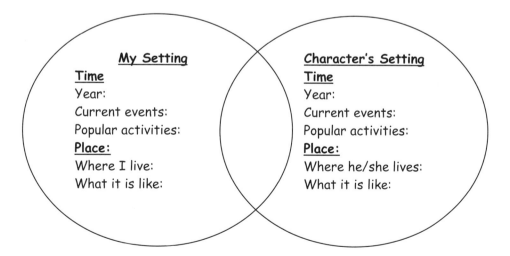

FIGURE 6.6. Structured Venn diagram to help students think flexibly about a story's setting.

dix 11). This graphic organizer can be used as a prewriting strategy for organizing paragraphs or essays. It encourages students to provide specific examples, and it also helps to ensure that the details support the argument and promote the main idea.

Another method for promoting flexible thinking when writing is to teach students to develop counterarguments to their theses or main ideas. Introducing a counterargument is an effective technique for an introduction or conclusion to a persuasive essay. Developing an introductory or concluding statement that challenges an argument, but is weighted more heavily in the direction of the writer's opinion, encourages a student to think deeply and flexibly about the topic at hand.

Note taking is another area of written language that requires students to think flexibly. When taking notes during a class lecture, students are required to listen actively to the information, transfer it into their own words, and record important information in note form. Similarly, effective note taking while reading requires students to read the information and paraphrase it in words that are meaningful and familiar to them. However, the act of paraphrasing is extremely challenging for many students, especially those who have difficulty thinking flexibly. As a result, these students frequently resort to copying the exact words that appear in the text; this not only compromises their understanding, but also reduces the likelihood that they will retain the information over time. Thus it is essential to provide students with explicit instruction focused on ways of paraphrasing information for note taking. The following four-step process for teaching paraphrasing is effective (Vener, 2002):

1. Find the words you want to change.
2. Use a thesaurus to find appropriate synonyms for these words.
3. Replace the original words with the synonyms.
4. Rearrange the sentence so that it makes sense, without changing its original meaning.

Teachers should also explain to students that their notes need to be legible and should contain accurate information, but that they do not have to use perfect spelling and grammar or to write in complete sentences. Instead, students can use bullets or numbers to take notes and can develop personalized systems of abbreviations for common words.

Shifting and Flexible Thinking in Math

In math, shifting is essential for efficient and accurate calculations and analyses of word problems. Students often need to shift flexibly between operations (e.g., long division involves shifting from division to multiplication to subtraction). Students are also often taught to predict the answers and generate estimates before solving problems. In other words, they need to shift flexibly between the initial "ballpark figure" or estimate and the actual answer. Moreover, when solving word problems, students often need to shift fluidly between numbers and words. For example, they need to know that the key phrase *all together* indicates addition, whereas the phrase *less than* calls for subtraction. When asked to "explain their work," students need to work in the opposite direction and convert their numerical computations into written language.

One way to promote flexible thinking in math is to expose students to multiple representations of mathematical concepts and procedures (Roditi & Steinberg, 2007). Many teachers already use multiple representations when teaching fractions, decimals, and percents, all of which can be expressed by using numbers, words, and visual or concrete manipulatives that illustrate part-to-whole relationships. To help students think flexibly about the concepts they are learning, this type of instruction can be extended to many more mathematical constructs. Positive and negative numbers, for example, can be illustrated by using a traditional number line or the analogy of temperature on a thermometer. Similarly, asking students to convert numbers into graphs, tables, and charts helps them to shift from the smaller details to the larger patterns and trends.

When learning new concepts or skills, students are frequently required to practice problems presented in a particular format in class or for homework. To promote mastery of mathematical skills, this format is often highly structured and repetitive. For tests or quizzes, teachers often change the format to evaluate their students' level of comprehension, in addition to their ability to apply these skills. Teachers may also group together different types of problems that students have previously practiced only in isolation. On these tasks, students often have difficulty shifting mindsets and recognizing familiar problems that are presented in a different format. They also struggle to differentiate between mixed problem types (see Figure 6.7).

Example 1: Calculation

Homework: What is 20 percent of 80?

Test: 16 is what percent of 80?

Example 2: Word Problem

Homework: John earns the following scores on his English tests: 82, 90, 76, and 87. What is his average test score for the semester?

Test: Rachel's average test score for the semester in history class is an 89. She earned the following scores on three of the tests: 92, 88, and 81. What score must she have earned on the fourth test?

FIGURE 6.7. Examples of math problems with different formats.

- Is this problem the same as or different from the one I did before?
- If it is different, *what* is different about it? For example, does it require a different operation or a different algorithm?
- What specific steps do I need to follow in order to solve *this* problem?

FIGURE 6.8. Suggestions for helping students to shift among problem types.

To address situations such as those in Figure 6.7, it is important to teach students how to shift flexibly from one problem type to another or one format to another. When completing a page of multiple problem types for homework or on a test, for example, students can be encouraged to stop and ask themselves the specific questions presented in Figure 6.8. These questions help them identify the similarities and differences between the problem they are currently working on and the previous problems in that set. These guided questions are intended to help students not to get "stuck" in one approach, but to shift flexibly in order to recognize the differences between problems. Students can then recognize that a different approach or operation may be needed and can generate a more accurate plan of action.

Shifting and Flexible Thinking for Studying and Taking Tests

As discussed above, preparing for tests and quizzes is a process that requires flexible thinking on many different levels. Students need to be able to extract information from a variety of sources, including textbooks, homework assignments, and class notes. Memorizing the specific details and integrating them with the larger concepts also require cognitive flexibility. Students with executive function difficulties often experience an overload of information, so that they do not know where to begin; as a result, they often feel as if their minds are like "clogged funnels" (see Figure 1.2 in Chapter 1). Because they do not shift approaches flexibly and cannot sift and sort the information, they cannot unclog their funnels easily. Consequently, their writing, study skills, and test performance are often compromised, and their academic grades often do not reflect their true intellectual ability.

Many students tend to use the same study techniques for all subject areas. Although it may be effective to focus on the textbook to prepare for a history test, this may be less helpful in math, where it is often more beneficial to review earlier classwork and homework assignments. Students need to be taught that different subject areas require different study techniques, and that they need to be flexible in their preparation for tests and quizzes. Helping students to develop a systematic study plan for each subject area, such as the one in Figure 6.9, is one way to

Math

Make a flash card for each different type of problem. Each card should include these details:

- Name of problem
- How to recognize it
- Steps to solve it
- Example
- Strategy for remembering the information

Make a practice test with examples of each type of problem.
Check work carefully. Redo the problems that were challenging or incorrect.

English

Write a one- or two-sentence summary of each chapter in the novel. Identify important examples and quotes from each chapter.

Review the notes from class.

Try to predict the essay question. Create an outline for a response.

FIGURE 6.9. Examples of personalized study plans for math and English.

help students recognize this. Students should develop individualized study plans reflecting the study strategies that have proved to be most effective for them.

Even within the same subject area, students should also be taught to study differently for tests with different formats. For a multiple-choice format test in history, students are often tested on detailed, factual information. For an essay test in history, however, students need to be taught how to shift away from the facts and details to the topics or major concepts. They need to be able to "tell the story" embedded in the content, rather than simply cramming hundreds of facts/details and then forgetting these immediately after the test.

For short-answer and essay tests, students are required to select the most relevant factual information and to connect these details to a larger theme. One effective study strategy for such tests is to review the textbook, class notes, and homework assignments, and them to make strategy notecards with important people, dates, places, and events on one side, and the corresponding descriptions on the other. Students should also write down their personalized strategies for remembering key terms and for shifting from the major concepts to the relevant details, such as a crazy phrases, acronyms, or cartoons (see Chapters 2 and 5 for more details). In fact, it is beneficial for students to create three-column notes, where they record the main idea in one column, the supporting details in a second column, and their memory strategies in the last column. The Triple Note Tote strategy from BrainCogs (ResearchILD & FableVision, 2003) can be used in this way for taking notes, outlining, studying, and self-quizzing (see Chapters 2, 4, and 5 for more information).

Helping Leo and Sally to Think More Flexibly

As demonstrated by the descriptions of Leo and Sally at the beginning of this chapter, students' difficulties in thinking flexibly can affect their learning and academic performance in a variety of ways. Therefore, it is important to select the techniques used to promote flexible thinking carefully, in order to match students' individual learning profiles and address their academic needs. Table 6.4 provides a few suggestions for helping Leo and Sally think more flexibly and for addressing their respective areas of difficulty: in math and science (Leo) and in language arts (Sally).

TABLE 6.4. Suggestions for Helping Leo and Sally to Think Flexibly

Difficulty	Recommendations
	Leo
Applying familiar information to new problems or situations presented on science and math quizzes and tests	• For novel problems, teach Leo to ask himself what is the same and what is different or new about this problem versus problems he has completed previously for homework. He should then use this information to create a plan of action. • Create a study plan for tests and quizzes, which includes having Leo practice applying the skills and information that he knows to new situations. Develop Leo's metacognitive awareness by providing explicit examples that emphasize cognitive flexibility. Provide opportunities for modeling, guided practice, and independent practice.
Shifting approaches when solving math problems	• Use multiple representations of information (e.g., algorithms, graphs, diagrams) to teach math concepts and skills. Make the connections between the different representations explicit and clear. • Develop Leo's metacognitive awareness by providing opportunities for him to reflect on his strategy use. Leo could be given extra credit for completing strategy reflection sheets for his homework or tests.
	Sally
Identifying the main ideas while reading and note-taking	• Teach Sally how to change subheadings into questions (see Chapters 4 and 5) to extract the main ideas from each section of her textbook. Encourage her to write down the answer on a Post-it Note that is stuck directly to the book, or to use a three-column note-taking format (see Chapters 4 and 5). • For note taking, Sally can paraphrase information and use a personalized system of abbreviations.
Shifting flexibly between the main idea (or thesis) and details in written language	• Before writing essays, Sally can use the STAR strategy (see Chapters 1 and 5) or the graphic organizer in Appendix 12, to ensure that the details and quotes she includes in her essay support her main idea. • When she studies for essay and short-answer tests, Sally can predict what the questions might be and make a draft or outline of her answers.

CONCLUSION

Cognitive flexibility, or the ability to think flexibly and to shift mindsets, is one of the least understood executive function processes. There is a need for many more studies that systematically evaluate the links between cognitive flexibility and performance in the different academic domains. It is important that teachers build time into the daily curriculum for teaching students to develop metacognitive mindsets and to think strategically about their work. Students need to learn why and how they can approach all academic tasks flexibly, so they can shift easily "from the top of the mountain to the bottom," as they focus alternately on the major themes and the relevant details (see Figure 1.1 in Chapter 1). In doing so, they learn to prioritize, to sift and sort information, and to "unclog the funnel" (see Figure 1.2 in Chapter 1) so that they can be productive and successful in school and in life.

CHAPTER 7

Self-Monitoring and Self-Checking

The Cornerstones of Independent Learning

JENNIFER SAGE BAGNATO and LYNN MELTZER

> I always remind Malcolm to check his work before handing it in.
> Even with these constant reminders, his work is filled with careless
> mistakes that could have been avoided if only he had proofread more
> carefully. In math, he seems to understand the concepts and is able to
> follow the steps of the procedures, but he frequently makes calculation
> errors that result in wrong answers. While his essays are organized
> and well developed, his grammar, punctuation and spelling are poor,
> which makes his writing difficult to understand. He puts a lot of time
> and effort into his writing, but his grades are still low.
>
> —NINTH-GRADE TEACHER

WHY ARE SELF-MONITORING AND SELF-CORRECTING SO IMPORTANT?

Self-monitoring refers to the ways in which learners manage their cognitive and metacognitive processes to track their own performance and outcomes (Zimmerman, 1998, 2000; Zimmerman & Kitsantas, 1997; Zimmerman & Schunk, 2001). When students self-monitor, they review their progress toward their goals, evaluate the outcomes, and redirect their efforts when needed. The ability to self-monitor depends on students' metacognitive awareness, as well as on their flexibility in shifting back and forth from the final product of their efforts to the goal of the tasks. Therefore, students' self-monitoring strategies relate to their ability to recognize when, how, and why to use specific strategies; to check the effectiveness of their strategy use; to evaluate and revise their strategy use; and to continually adjust their use of strategies based on the task demands. This chapter is limited to a discussion of self-monitoring and self-checking strategies, and does not address the broader topic of self-regulation or the range of definitions and theoretical models that have evolved within the cognitive, behavioral, social, and educational domains (Graham & Harris, 2003). Many of the strategies discussed here are based on clinical studies or school-based studies that have assessed the efficacy of clusters of executive function strategies, rather than focusing on individual self-checking strategies. These suggestions are provided as a framework that teachers can use to guide their approaches as they encourage their students to stop, reflect on their work, and develop their own personalized self-checking strategies.

Students with learning and attention problems often have difficulty with monitoring their own learning, as well as evaluating the connections among their effort, strategy use, and performance. As they focus their effort on reading, writing, math problem solving, and content learning, they may struggle to monitor their attention and performance, and may have difficulty shifting among the various problem-solving approaches or strategies that are available to them (Klingner, Vaughn, & Boardman, 2007; Montague, 2003). These students need systematic, structured, and scaffolded instruction in using self-monitoring strategies flexibly, so that they can become independent learners who do not need the assistance of others to complete reading, writing, math, or other academic tasks successfully (Graham & Harris, 2003; Reid & Lienemann, 2006). Systematic teaching of these self-monitoring strategies is beneficial for all students, but it is essential for students with learning and attention problems (Meltzer et al., 2001, 2004a).

Students with *intrinsic* motivation and *growth* mindsets (Dweck, 2006; Dweck & Molden, 2005) usually set learning goals for themselves and focus on learning as much as possible for the sake of learning. They also use self-regulatory strategies to sustain their motivation and make the effort to monitor, check, revise, and correct their own work (Dweck & Molden, 2004). Students with extrinsic motivation and fixed mindsets (Dweck, 2006; Dweck & Molden, 2004) usually set performance goals (e.g., obtaining high grades) and do not easily shift approaches or use strategies to revise their work. These students believe that if they need to work harder and expend more effort, this indicates that they are not very smart and lack ability (Dweck & Molden, 2004). Therefore, teachers need to recognize that their classes are very likely to include students with both types of mindsets. Consequently, the classroom culture needs to value the importance of the learning process, or the *how* of learning. Similarly, students need to understand the emphasis teachers place on effort, as well as strategies for self-monitoring and revising. When the classroom culture fosters growth mindsets, as well as persistence and effort, students with fixed mindsets whose goals center around higher grades are forced to shift and recognize the importance of effort, as well as strategies for checking, editing, and revising their work (Elliot & Dweck, 2005).

In this chapter, we discuss *how* to teach students self-monitoring strategies, as well as *what* specific strategies can be taught in the classroom to help students to check and correct their own work systematically. There is an emphasis on the important role of cognitive flexibility in the self-checking process, and strategies are discussed that help students to shift back and forth between the product and the process. These strategies enable students to recognize that learning is dynamic and constantly evolves and changes. The links between these self-monitoring strategies and the executive function processes discussed in previous chapters—namely, goal setting, planning, prioritizing, organizing, memorizing, and thinking flexibly/shifting mindsets—are also addressed. Again, the suggestions in this chapter are provided as a broad guide for teachers, so that they have a foundation for developing and embedding their own approaches and strategies within their classroom curricula.

HOW CAN WE TEACH STUDENTS TO USE SELF-MONITORING AND SELF-CHECKING STRATEGIES?

The most effective self-monitoring and self-checking approaches involve what Harris and Graham (1996) refer to as *self-assessment* and *self-recording*. Students need to know the expectations of an assignment, as well as the criteria and standards by which it will be evaluated, so that they can compare their performance to these standards and can record their personal progress on a checklist or chart. They also need to learn what types of errors to check for, how to recognize their most common errors, and how to revise their work to be successful (Graham, MacArthur, & Fitzgerald, 2007; Harris & Graham, 1996; Maccini & Hughes, 1997; Mastropieri & Scruggs, 1995). For example, when completing math calculations, students with attention problems who often rush and make impulsive errors can slow themselves down by highlighting the operations in each problem and using a different method to check the calculations. For word problems, students can first estimate the answer to each problem, and then compare the estimate to the answer to evaluate whether or not their answer makes sense. Furthermore, students can record the number of errors they make on a daily checklist and graph their errors each day. This self-assessment helps students to visually monitor their performance, to observe the frequency of their errors, and to take control over the learning process.

In this regard, numerous studies have shown that teaching self-monitoring strategies systematically to students with learning disabilities can improve their performance significantly (Graham & Harris, 2003; Harris & Graham, 1996; Reid, 1996; Reid & Harris, 1993; Shimabukuro, Prater, Jenkins, & Edelen-Smith, 1999; Webber, Scheuermann, McCall, & Coleman, 1993). Furthermore, harnessing students' interest in the content of complex reading material often improves their use of strategies and engagement, as they are more willing to ponder and persist with demanding domain tasks (Alexander, 2004; Alexander & Murphy, 1998). Structured classroom environments and systematic approaches to teaching strategies can increase students' willingness to shift approaches and make the extra effort to use self-checking strategies.

Explicit, structured, systematic teaching is critically important for improving students' understanding of their learning profiles and increasing their willingness to slow down and take the necessary time to spiral back and forth between the task demands and their own output (Meltzer et al., 2007b; Reid & Lienemann, 2006). For example, when students are given a word problem to solve in math, they benefit from a comprehensive instructional routine such as Montague's Solve It! (Montague, Warger, & Morgan, 2000). This routine teaches them how to read the problem for understanding, paraphrase by putting the problem into their own words, visualize the problem by drawing a picture or making a mental image, set up a plan for solving the problem, estimate the answer, compute, and check to verify the solution. Students also need to be taught the self-regulation strategies needed for effective math problem solving, which include giving themselves instructions, asking themselves questions as they go through the problem-solving steps, and monitoring their performance (Meltzer & Montague, 2001; Montague, 2003; Montague et al., 2000). These examples of explicit and systematic instruction help problem solvers gain access to strategic knowledge, apply strategies, and regulate their use of strategies and overall performance as they solve complex problems.

Students often feel overwhelmed by the enormous volume of information they are required to learn and the many subskills they need to coordinate simultaneously. As a result, they have trouble shifting to a self-checking mindset, and do not stop to look for possible errors and to revise their work. As discussed in Chapter 1, teachers can help students to self-monitor and self-correct by teaching them to visualize themselves standing at the "top of the mountain" (e.g., in their writing, focusing on the "big picture" or main ideas) then shifting to the "bottom of the mountain" (e.g., focusing on the details to check for spelling, tenses, etc.), and then shifting back to the top again. Furthermore, teachers can help students to continually prioritize, organize, and reorganize complex information, so that their executive function strategies can keep the "funnel unclogged" and the large volume of information flowing through the funnel (again, see Chapter 1). Teachers can also help students to visualize the shifts they need to make between major ideas and details by using analogies, such as a zoom lens on a camera zoom.

It is important for teachers to teach a range of self-monitoring/self-correcting approaches systematically, and to provide time on a daily basis for students to implement and evaluate these strategies. When teachers make these strategies count by grading students on their use in classwork, homework, and tests, the students are more likely to value the strategies and to use them consistently (Meltzer et al., 2004a, 2004b, 2004c; Meltzer et al., 2007b).

How Can Teachers Create a Classroom Culture Where Students Self-Monitor and Self-Check?

The following suggestions may be helpful for teachers and can be adapted to the needs of different groups of students:

1. Help students develop their own daily checklists to remind them to complete their homework, bring their homework to school, and hand their assignments to their teachers.
2. Encourage students to tape prompts to their lockers, so they remember to take the correct books and assignments to each class and the appropriate materials home for homework.
3. Help students to internalize the reasons for their successes or failures appropriately. Attribute successes to their hard work and appropriate use of strategies, and failures to their lack of strategy use rather than lack of ability (Elliot & Dweck, 2005).
4. Base feedback to students on their strategy use and effort, rather than on their final answers to questions.
5. Teach students how to shift mindsets and approaches so they can identify *and* correct their errors.
6. Make self-monitoring and self-correcting requirements rather than options.
7. Make self-monitoring and self-checking *count*! Require students to use strategy reflection sheets to list the strategies they have used in their homework and on tests (see Chapters 1 and 2).
8. Give students bonus points or credit toward their grades for finding and fixing mistakes on homework assignments and tests.
9. Allow students to refer to their strategy notecards and personalized error checklists during tests.
10. Give students additional time on tests to check and correct their work.
11. Provide students with additional credit if they show evidence of using checking strategies.
12. Introduce students to ideas that help them to switch to a self-checking mindset and to focus their attention on the self-checking process. Examples of ideas that have been helpful in clinical settings, but are not yet evidence-based, include the following:
    - *Shifting materials.* Give students concrete cues that can help them switch to a learning mindset (e.g., students can switch from one pen or pencil to another with a different grip or color when they check their work).
    - *Shifting the medium.* For example, encourage students to change from the computer to a hard copy in order to check and correct work.
    - *Shifting from silent to oral reading.* Encourage students to read a written piece aloud, so that they have oral cues to help them identify and correct their errors.

WHAT SPECIFIC STRATEGIES SHOULD BE TAUGHT TO HELP STUDENTS SELF-MONITOR AND SELF-CHECK SYSTEMATICALLY?

Self-Monitoring/Self-Checking Strategies for Reading

Individual Word Reading

Reading is a complex process that requires continuous self-monitoring and cognitive flexibility on many levels. For individual word reading, it is helpful to teach students to monitor and be mindful of the strategies they use to read unfamiliar words. Once they are aware of the strategies they are using to read, they can select and apply these strategies more flexibly. Thus a student whose initial attempt at word reading is unsuccessful can try a different approach and choose an alternative strategy, rather than "getting stuck."

SELF-MONITORING WORD READING

Through modeling, guided practice, and explicit instruction, students can be introduced to different word-reading strategies, including recognizing words by sight, decoding (or "sounding out"), applying knowledge of word morphology (such as prefixes and suffixes), and using context clues embedded in the sentence (Combs, 1996). It is also important to emphasize that a combination of strategies may be used to read a single word. When readers encounter an unknown word, they can be encouraged to reflect on the strategies they used to read it and write the symbols above the text, as shown in Figure 7.1.

Symbol	Word-Reading Strategy
	Did I recognize the word right away?
	Did I sound it out?
	Did I pull it apart?
	Did I use other clues in the sentence?

FIGURE 7.1. Self-monitoring word reading.

Click and Clunk

Click and Clunk (Klingner & Vaughn, 1996) is another self-monitoring strategy to help students monitor their comprehension at the word level. This is a key element of the evidence-based *collaborative strategic reading* approach developed by Klingner and Vaughn (1996). Students are encouraged to "click and clunk" as they read; a *click* is described as text that they read fluently and understand, whereas a *clunk* refers to text that is confusing or unknown. When students encounter clunks in the text, they are encouraged to use clunk cards with strategies for figuring out the meanings of the unfamiliar words. The strategies include rereading the sentence with the clunk and looking for context clues; rereading the sentences before and after the clunk; looking for context clues; pulling apart the words; and looking for prefixes, suffixes, and familiar word parts (Bremer, Vaughn, Clapper, & Kim, 2002).

Comprehension of Fiction

In addition to monitoring reading at the word level, students must be taught how to monitor their comprehension at the sentence and paragraph levels. Various strategies may be used to encourage students to use more systematic and active approaches for checking their understanding at these levels when they are reading fiction.

MARGIN NOTES

When reading a novel, students can be asked to write margin notes in response to the text. To do so, students are given a key with symbols that correspond to specific responses to the text (see Figure 7.2 for an example). If they encounter something surprising in the reading, they put an exclamation mark next to that section of the text. If they come across a word or section of the text that they did not understand, they are encouraged to write a question mark in the margin. This shorthand approach to note taking helps students monitor their comprehension and reactions to the text while reading. It also provides them with notes to refer to when they are asked to write about or discuss the novel after reading. Over time, students should be encouraged to create their own symbols and to develop a personalized system for writing margin notes.

Symbol	Response for text that is . . .
!	Surprising
?	Confusing
☺	Interesting or fun to read
**	Important to remember

FIGURE 7.2. Sample key for writing margin notes in narrative text.

SUMMARY POST-IT NOTES

Another way to encourage students to monitor their comprehension of a novel is to have them write a short summary at the end of each chapter on a lined Post-it Note. Post-it Notes are helpful organizational tools, as they can be stuck to the last page of each chapter. They are easily accessible for students who need to review continuously what has happened in the novel. To write effective summary notes, students need to be taught, through modeling and explicit instruction, how to identify the main events of a chapter.

Comprehension of Informational Text

Comprehending informational text can be challenging for students on many levels. As they often have difficulty processing the volume of information presented in one page, it can be overwhelming for them to organize this information in a meaningful way. As a result, students typically skim the reading or ignore it altogether. When they are asked to answer the review questions at the end of the chapter, some students often scour the pages to find the answers, leaving them with a very superficial and piecemeal understanding of the topic. To facilitate a more thorough and holistic understanding, students need to be taught how to engage in the text and self-monitor their comprehension.

CHANGING SECTION HEADINGS INTO QUESTIONS

Using a science or social studies textbook as an example, students can learn about the underlying structure of a textbook, so that they can easily identify a section heading. They can then practice turning section headings into questions. (For example, a section titled "Causes of the Revolutionary War" would become "What Were the Causes of the Revolutionary War?"). Once they have mastered these skills, students can be required to read each section, turn the heading into a question, and provide the response either on a Post-it Note that can be stuck to the textbook or on a separate piece of paper. This systematic approach not only helps students to monitor their understanding of the text as they read, but also helps them to organize the information and extract the main idea from each section.

Self-Monitoring/Self-Checking Strategies for Written Language

As part of the writing process, teachers commonly encourage students to edit their writing. However, many students have difficulty actually seeing their mistakes. Thus, when students are checking their work, it is essential to teach them how to shift mindsets from that of the "writer" to that of the "editor." As discussed above, this shift may be facilitated by having students use a different-colored pencil or pen to edit their work; read their written work aloud; or, if they wrote the original draft on a computer, print it out and edit a hard copy.

As students often have difficulty knowing what to look for in their writing, it is also important that they be given explicit direction about *what* to edit. A "one size fits all," generic editing checklist is often not effective, because different students make different types of mistakes in their writing. For instance, one student may consistently make spelling errors but have no difficulty with organization; another may have the opposite profile. When they are provided with explicit checklists for particular assignments, students will know what to check for and will make fewer errors. As demonstrated by Graham and Harris (2005), for example, providing students with a checklist that outlines the main elements of a narrative story, (e.g., setting, character, conflict, resolution) helps students to produce better-developed and higher-quality narratives. While they are planning and writing, students are taught to use these checklists to self-monitor, whether or not they have incorporated important story parts. The same approach may be used for persuasive writing. Here students are taught to monitor their inclusion of the basic structural components of persuasive writing: topic sentence, reasons, refutations, examples, and endings (Graham, 1990).

Personalized Editing Checklists

Students should be encouraged to analyze several of their writing samples to determine their most common mistakes. From this, they can develop a personalized editing checklist that directs them to check for these errors. Figure 7.3 provides one example of a personalized checklist developed by an elementary school teacher for her students.

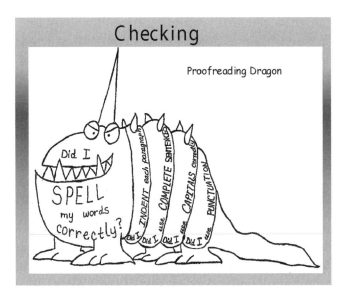

FIGURE 7.3. Personalized editing checklist for early elementary school.

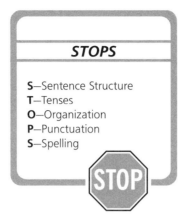

FIGURE 7.4. STOPS: A personalized editing checklist for upper elementary and middle school levels. Developed by Colin Meltzer, 1995. From Meltzer, Sales Pollica, and Barzillai (2007b). Copyright 2007 by The Guilford Press. Reprinted by permission.

It is often helpful for students to develop an acronym to help them remember what to look for in their writing. The acronym STOPS, for example, was developed by a sixth grader to cue him to check his writing for errors he commonly made: namely, problems with sentence structure, consistent use of verb tenses (i.e., he tended to mix present, past, and future tenses), organization of ideas, punctuation, and spelling.

Guide for Making Revisions

In addition to editing for mechanical errors, students are usually asked to revise their work in order to improve its content, structure, and organization. Typically, students are given a rubric that outlines the expectations for the assignment in these areas. However, they often have difficulty interpreting the rubric and evaluating whether their writing meets the criteria. Even if they recognize that their writing is below expectations in a certain category, they often do not know how to make the necessary improvements. Thus, to help students revise their written work more effectively, they need to be given tools that help them know *what* to improve and *how* to improve it. An essay revision guide is provided in Appendix 12. This not only helps students to evaluate their writing with respect to content, structure, and organization, but also provides them with guidance for making changes.

Self-Monitoring/Self-Checking Strategies for Math

Students are often reminded to check their math work after they finish a homework assignment or test. Yet, as with writing, they have difficulty finding their math errors and making the necessary corrections. As a result, even students who possess a strong conceptual understanding of mathematical skills or procedures often make careless errors that significantly diminish their performance. When checking their work, students need to be reminded to shift mindsets from the "math problem solver" to the "math checker." Again, encouraging students to check their math work with a different-colored pen or pencil is a symbolic way to represent this shift.

Error Analysis

Similar to the personalized checklists described in the writing section above, math checklists can help students analyze their math work to determine the kinds of mistakes they tend to make. For each unit, they can be given a list of very specific, common errors that they often make when applying this skill. The checklist in Figure 7.5, for example, would be appropriate for a unit on multiplication and division of fractions. It helps students to calculate, categorize, and see patterns in their mistakes.

Once students are aware of the kinds of mistakes they tend to make when carrying out a particular operation or procedure, they can use this information to develop a personalized checklist, along with a crazy phrase or other mnemonic to help them remember the strategy (see Chapter 5 for more specific memory strategies). Writing their checklist at the top of their homework page or test will help them to remember what to look for when checking their work.

Analysis of Test Performance

In addition to reading each individual problem to determine where an error may have occurred, students should be encouraged to use a more "macro" view when analyzing their test performance. This is especially true for students who seem to understand the mathematical skills and concepts in class and on their homework, but have difficulty showing what they know on tests and quizzes. In this case, students can be given a guide for analyzing their test performance, such as the one in Figure 7.6.

Type of Problem	Possible Errors	Number of Errors
×	Didn't multiply horizontally (across)	0
÷	Didn't invert the numerator and denominator	2
× and ÷	Didn't simplify the answer	4
× and ÷	Didn't multiply the numbers correctly	0

FIGURE 7.5. Sample guide for analyzing errors in multiplying and dividing fractions.

Performance Area	Number of Errors	Percentage of Total Errors*
Directions	0	0%
Vocabulary	6	35%
Concept	2	12%
Calculation	8	47%
Attention to detail	1	<6%

*Calculated by dividing the number of errors in each category by the total number of errors.

FIGURE 7.6. Sample guide for analyzing test performance.

Quantifying and categorizing their errors will help students to see patterns in their mistakes. Most importantly, such analysis will also help focus their approach to preparing and studying for the next test. The student whose test performance is analyzed in Figure 7.6, for example, clearly needs to focus on learning the math vocabulary more effectively and calculating more accurately.

Word Problem Analysis

In addition to checking their work while performing calculations, students need to check their work carefully while solving problems. Problem solving is difficult for many students, because it requires them to integrate a variety of skills and to complete multiple steps. Word problems are especially challenging, as they require students to shift flexibly between numbers and words. Because there are so many opportunities for errors to occur, it is important for students to utilize a consistent, reliable, and systematic strategy for checking their work. To help improve students' accuracy and efficiency while solving word problems, they can be encouraged to implement the steps below and ask themselves the following questions:

- Read: Did I read the question carefully?
- Circle: Did I circle the keywords and relevant numbers?
- Estimate: Did I estimate the answer?
- Calculate: Did I calculate correctly?
- Compare: Did I compare my estimate to my answer? Is my answer reasonable?
- Possible crazy phrases: Rowdy Chimps Enjoy Checkers and Chess, Ravenous Chickens Eat Crunchy Cheerios.

Following the steps above, students are first cued to read the question carefully and restate it in their own words. Next, they circle key words and relevant numbers, estimate the answer, and then perform the necessary calculation(s). For the final step, students are taught to compare their estimate to their answer—an important step in helping students to self-monitor their work. If their final answer is reasonable and close to their initial estimate, students know that they are on the right track. However, if the final answer differs significantly from the estimate, then it is likely that a mistake was made along the way.

Self-Monitoring/Self-Checking Strategies for Test Taking

Teachers regularly remind students to check their work before handing in tests. However, most students, especially those who tend to make many careless mistakes, need explicit instruction on what to look for and how to check their work. Below are examples of strategies to help students check their work more carefully and systematically.

Checking Cards

Laminated test-checking cards can be given to each student at the beginning of the year (see Appendix 13). While reviewing their tests, students can be reminded to refer to their checking cards. Over time, students can be encouraged to develop personalized test-checking cards that cue them to look for the mistakes they tend to make. Ultimately, by using the cards consistently, students will internalize the checking process. This makes it more likely that they will initiate checking on their own, without being prompted, so that it becomes an automatic step in their test-taking process. Checking cards may be especially helpful for visual and "hands-on" learners.

Crazy Phrases

For students who learn more easily when information is presented verbally rather than visually, it may be helpful to encourage them to develop a crazy phrase that cues them to look for the errors they tend to make on tests. "Never Drink Sour Coffee," for example, is a crazy phrase that reminds students to check the following:

- Name: Did I write my name on the test?
- Directions: Did I follow the directions?
- Strategies: Did I use my strategies?
- Corrections: Did I check my work and make corrections?

Strategies to Help Malcolm Self-Monitor and Self-Check

As described by his teacher in the quotation at the start of this chapter, Malcolm, like many students, has difficulty self-monitoring his performance. His perfor-

TABLE 7.1. Self-Monitoring/Self-Checking Strategies to Help Malcolm with His Work

Difficulty	Recommendations
Identifying and correcting careless mistakes in math	• Encourage Malcolm to analyze his past math quizzes/tests and homework assignments, to identify his common math mistakes. Use this error analysis to develop a personalized math checklist.
	• Encourage Malcolm to use a different-colored pencil for checking his math work.
	• Teach Malcolm to use a systematic approach to word problems, such as Read, Circle, Estimate, Calculate, Compare (see text). Comparing his answer to his estimate will help Malcolm to evaluate whether or not his answer makes sense and to recognize when a miscalculation may have occurred.
Recognizing and correcting errors in writing	• Encourage Malcolm to analyze his writing and to identify his most common mistakes. Develop an individualized writing checklist for proofreading.
	• Encourage Malcolm to read his written work aloud when proofreading and/or to use a different-colored pencil when checking.
	• Give Malcolm a revision guide for essays (see Appendix 12), to help him evaluate his writing and to provide suggestions for improving his written work.
Identifying and correcting errors while taking quizzes and tests	• Require Malcolm to analyze his past tests and quizzes, to identify his test-taking strengths and weaknesses. Being aware of his common mistakes will help him to study more effectively and know what details to check on tests.
	• Encourage Malcolm to develop a crazy phrase that cues him to look for the errors he tends to make on tests, such as "Never Drink Sour Coffee" (Name, Directions, Strategies, and Corrections).
	• Allow Malcolm to use checking cards for quizzes and tests.
	• Award Malcolm bonus points or credit toward his grade for finding and fixing mistakes on quizzes and tests.

mance in math and written work is affected by his inattention to details, and he makes many careless mistakes that he cannot identify. Table 7.1 provides examples of specific strategies to help Malcolm self-monitor and self-correct his academic performance more effectively. All these strategies have been discussed previously in this chapter.

CONCLUSION

Effective self-monitoring and self-checking require students to reflect on their progress toward a predetermined goal, to select strategies that are working, and to alter strategies that are not working. Many students with learning and attention difficulties have trouble with these processes, and thus their classroom performance is characterized by many careless mistakes, inefficient use of strategies, and difficulty seeing tasks through to completion. Despite frequent reminders from teachers and parents to "check their work," they do not know *what* to look for or *how* to edit their work. As a result, they make only minimal changes, if any. Explicit and systematic self-monitoring and self-correcting strategies, such as those described in this chapter, help students to develop their metacognitive awareness and improve their ability to evaluate their progress toward meeting a goal. The overall quality of their academic work improves when they are able to recognize the value of reviewing their work and shifting mindsets, so that they can stand at the "top of the mountain" to check the major themes and then shift flexibly to the "bottom of the mountain" to check the details (see Chapter 1). As Chapter 8 makes clear, students' motivation and emotional mindsets often affect their willingness to make the often superhuman effort needed to stop, reflect, check, and correct multiple drafts of their work—executive function processes that are critically important for academic and life success.

CHAPTER 8

Emotional Self-Regulation

A Critical Component of Executive Function

JUDITH A. STEIN

Jacob, a 13-year-old seventh grader, proudly presents his original rap song, which he spent many hours creating for a social studies project. Another student sings a well-known song to the class for her project. When his teacher gives Jacob a lower grade on the assignment than she does to the second student, Jacob is devastated and infuriated. As a result, he withdraws from the teacher and loses interest in the class. For the rest of the year, his motivation, his effort, and the quality of his work decline precipitously.

Jessica, an 11-year-old fifth grader, has always struggled with math. She is unable to pass the "mad minute" multiplication tests that are given every Friday. At the end of each week, she is flooded with worry, often has a stomachache, and is on the verge of tears. No matter how hard she studies the night before, she cannot remember her multiplication facts. In fact, her math test scores have steadily declined throughout the year.

Rachel, a 15-year-old ninth grader, works hard to do well on every test. Because earning a high grade is so important to her, she becomes very anxious before every exam. Despite her long hours of preparation, Rachel often "freezes" when she sees a question or problem on a test for which she does not know the answer. At times, her mind goes blank and she is unable to finish the exam.

In each of these situations, students' difficulties in managing their emotional reactions to school-related events have dramatically negative effects on their academic performance. Like these students, many children and adolescents struggle with the stresses and the emotional ups and downs associated with the academic and social demands they face at school. As many as 17% of young people in the United States suffer from learning, emotional, or behavioral disorders that underlie their difficulties with emotional regulation (O'Connell, Boat, & Warner, 2009). In addition, many more students may have difficulty with emotional regulation when they are faced with stressful situations at home or school, such as illness, divorce, academic failure, or social isolation (Vail, 1994). In particular, students with learning and attention difficulties are at risk for becoming overly frustrated or anxiety-ridden by challenging academic tasks (Hallowell & Ratey, 1994; Rourke, 1995). At the middle and high school levels, some students may even "shut down" when their resources for regulating their emotions are depleted or overwhelmed (Goldstein & Brooks, 2005).

In this chapter, I discuss the components of emotional regulation, its importance as an executive function process, and its relationship to the other core executive function processes discussed in this book. A theoretical framework for understanding emotional regulation is presented, as well as specific strategies that teachers and other professionals can use to help their students develop more effective ways of managing their emotions and behavior. It should be noted, however, that a detailed discussion of impulse control and behavioral regulations is beyond the scope of this chapter. Most of the suggested strategies and interventions in this chapter have been widely used in both clinical and educational settings and have been found to be effective with specific students or in particular classrooms. Some of the recommended practices are evidence-based (i.e., their effectiveness has been substantiated by findings from experimental research), whereas others are based on clinical evidence or best practice. Those interventions that have been empirically supported are denoted as such in the discussion.

WHY IS EMOTIONAL REGULATION SO CRUCIAL
FOR ACADEMIC SUCCESS?

Mental health clinicians, researchers, and educators have long recognized that students' ability to regulate their emotions (and emotion-driven behavior) is an important factor that contributes to effective learning in a classroom environment (Brooks, 1991; Tangney, Baumeister, & Boone, 2004). The evidence accumulated by the expansion of brain-based research and neuroimaging studies has supported the observations of generations of teachers that children's capacity to pay attention for sufficient periods of time, engage actively in educational activities, and sustain their effort and motivation to tackle challenging tasks is associated with their level of emotional development (Gross, 2007). Success in the classroom depends upon students' ability to manage their emotions in appropriate ways. Either excessive displays of emotion or overly controlled affect can disrupt or impair the quality of teacher–student communication as well as interactions among peers. Emotional responses at either end of the continuum can also have a negative impact on the acquisition of new information, retrieval of learned material, and creative problem solving within the classroom.

A growing number of studies have found that levels of emotional arousal, as well as positive and negative mood states, affect brain functions that are critical for academic performance; these include attention, concentration, memory, and other executive function processes, such as inhibition, shifting, and strategy use (Begley, 2007; Gross, 2007; Phillips, Bull, Adams, & Fraser, 2002). Cognitive scientists and psychologists have shown that moderate levels of anxiety optimize performance on many tasks, such as oral presentations, competitive activities, and test taking. On the other hand, high levels of anxiety often impair concentration, memory, language, organization, and impulse control (Begley, 2007; Goleman, 1995). Negative moods have also been found to disrupt attention, concentration, memory, and processing speed. Although positive moods are reportedly beneficial for some cognitive processes, such as creative problem solving, they can also diminish specific executive function processes, such as planning, set shifting, and the retrieval of information (Gross, 2007). One explanation provided by Phillips et al. (2002) is that both negative and positive mood states can lead to distractions and thereby decrease students' concentration and ultimate efficiency in performing a complex task. Therefore, in order to optimize their learning in the classroom, students need to be aware of their emotions and to use effective self-regulatory strategies.

Students' emotional states and their success in regulating their emotions have a significant impact on their cognitive functioning, especially in the areas of planning, organizing, self-monitoring, and shifting. In turn, students who have difficulty with these executive function processes are often emotionally vulnerable (Stein & Krishnan, 2007). For example, some students with attention-deficit/hyperactivity disorder (ADHD) or nonverbal learning disabilities are easily frustrated, overwhelmed, and flooded with anxiety (Hallowell & Ratey, 1994; Rourke, 1995). One way of conceptualizing the interconnecting relationships between emotional regulation and other executive function processes is illustrated in Figure 8.1. All these processes are interdependent and can influence, as well as be influenced by, one another.

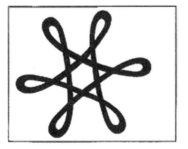

Emotional regulation

Goal setting/planning/prioritizing

Organizing

Accessing working memory

Self-monitoring/self-checking

Shifting/thinking flexibly

FIGURE 8.1. The interlocking relationship of emotional regulation to other executive function processes.

WHAT IS EMOTIONAL REGULATION?

Researchers and theorists have proposed various definitions of *emotional regulation*. Although most scientists agree that emotional regulation involves the internal processes by which an individual experiences an emotion, maintains it, and/or modifies it, there is some controversy concerning its definition. Some theorists, who take a broader view of this concept, include in their definition such factors as (1) the antecedents to emotional experience (e.g., personality traits, emotional well-being, and previous experiences); (2) the behaviors that are triggered by emotions; and (3) any external controls imposed by others to enhance self-regulation (Bridges, Margie, & Zaff, 2001; Gross, 2007; Macklem, 2008). For example, Macklem (2008) describes the process of emotional regulation as all of the actions an individual might take to control which emotions are experienced, how and when they are felt, and the ways in which they are expressed. Other theorists, who take a narrower view, focus primarily on the emotional changes that occur when an individual is affected by a specific event (Cole, Martin, & Dennis, 2004).

For the purposes of this chapter, *emotional regulation* is defined rather broadly as a multifaceted, complex process in which each individual's experience and expression of emotions are self-controlled (either consciously or unconsciously) or controlled by others (intentionally or unintentionally) (Gross, 2007). The ability to delay, fine-tune, modify, or shift one's emotions comprises an important and distinct executive function process (Hongwanishkul, Happaney, Lee, & Zelazo, 2005). The skill sets involved in emotional regulation include the ability to recognize and label one's own emotions, to understand one's emotional triggers, to manage the intensity of one's emotions, and to know when and how to express one's emotions in various social contexts. According to Gross (1998), emotional regulation can be understood as a series of five steps: (1) situation selection (the ability to interpret the context one encounters); (2) situation modification (the ability to use one's thinking and problem-solving ability to change the emotional impact of the situation); (3) attentional deployment (the ability to shift one's focus from the emotional trigger); (4) cognitive change (the ability to use one's thinking to reinterpret the situation and thus change one's emotional response); and (5) response modulation (the ability to use strategies to diminish the emotions one feels at the time).

Emotional responses can be modified along multiple dimensions, including timing, intensity, duration, and behavior (Gross & Thompson, 2007). Gross and Thompson's model further delineates the steps involved in the formation and modulation of emotions (see Figure 8.2). According to this model, emotions

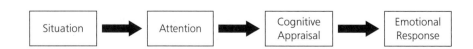

FIGURE 8.2. A model of emotional regulation. Based on Gross and Thompson (2007).

develop when an individual pays attention to a situation that is relevant to him or her, attributes a positive or negative meaning to the situation, and then responds accordingly. An emotional response encompasses a person's subjective experience, physiological reaction, and behavior. This response cycle is a recursive and flexible one, in that the emotional experience and expression change as the situation unfolds and/or the meaning of the situation shifts. The triggering event can either be an interaction occurring in the environment or an internal experience (e.g., a sensation, thought, image, or memory).

An individual's previous experiences, family and cultural background, emotional well-being, and many other variables affect which situations may trigger an emotional response. According to many social-cognitive theorists, an individual's emotional and behavioral reaction to a situation will in part be determined by the models the person has observed, as well as the reinforcement he or she has experienced in the past (Bandura, 1986; Dweck, 2006). Temperament and other personality characteristics, the presence or absence of an emotional or behavioral disorder, and previous conditioning will also influence what events and what circumstances will elicit a flood of emotions. In Gross and Thompson's model of emotional regulation, these factors, often known as *antecedents*, are reflected in the appraisal stage. In other words, how a person perceives and interprets an event encompasses all the antecedents and related factors that shape his or her appraisal of the situation.

The Development of Emotional Self-Regulation

Like other components of executive function, the emotional domain develops through the lifespan of the individual, beginning during the preschool period (Hongwanishkul et al., 2005).

Preschoolers begin to accumulate a fund of knowledge about the range of emotions, the recognition and names of basic feelings, the skills for modulating their feelings, and the appropriate ways to express their feelings within the cultural context of their environment (Stegge & Terwogt, 2007). As children mature, their ability to reflect on their own and others' feelings becomes more sophisticated and enables them to respond in a more flexible and adaptive manner. By the age of 6 years or so, children understand that emotional responses are related to their own internal beliefs and intentions, as well as to aspects of the triggering events. For example, if Jennifer believes that Emily is a friend, she will be kind and friendly toward her even if Emily really dislikes Jennifer. In the early elementary grades, however, children's understanding of aspects of their emotions is still somewhat simplistic. For instance, many 6-year-olds believe that their reactions to emotionally charged situations involve only one emotion, rather than the multiple emotions that may be elicited by a single interaction. Moreover, with respect to modifying their emotions, early elementary students are likely to believe that if they want to feel better in a distressing situation, they will need to change the situation in some way or refocus their attention on something else. They are unlikely to understand that they can alter their views of the situation or their emotional responses (Stegge & Terwogt, 2007).

By the time children reach the age of 10 years, they understand that they can experience multiple and sometimes conflicting feelings in a given situation. They also develop the ability to adjust their emotions according to the standards or cultural norms of their environment. For example, a child who gives an incorrect answer to a teacher's question may feel mildly uncomfortable or extremely embarrassed, depending on the teacher's expectations as well as on peers' reactions. As their mastery of emotional regulation grows, many children understand that it is important to disguise or withhold their feelings in certain situations. For instance, a student who is asked to evaluate a peer's project will understand that he or she should not express negative feelings about it. Furthermore, in the preadolescent period, children learn to regulate their negative feelings by understanding the situation from a different perspective (i.e., reappraising the situation) or finding an effective solution to the set of circumstances (Stegge & Terwogt, 2007). Table 8.1 summarizes the sequence in which emotional self-regulation develops.

Variability in Emotional Regulation

Although many children develop some competence in the area of emotional regulation by the early elementary grades, a significant number of children may be lagging in the development of this executive function process (Cole et al., 2004). Variations in emotional regulation among children may be due to a number of factors, including differences in age, genetics, temperament, parenting style, maturity, and cultural norms (Hongwanishkul et al., 2005; John & Gross, 2007; Zelazo et al., 2003). Some children may be genetically predisposed to experiencing heightened anxiety, irritability, depression, and impulsivity (Kagan, 1989; Ruf, Goldsmith, Lemery-Chalfant, & Schmidt, 2008; Tsai, Levenson, & McCox, 2006). In some cases, temperamental differences among children may account for various levels of emotional control, since one component of temperament is the intensity with which emotions are felt and expressed (Thomas & Chess, 1977). Still other children may

TABLE 8.1. Development of Emotional Self-Regulation

Ages	Skills
Preschool (3–5) years	Recognition and identification of feelings; an emerging understanding of appropriate ways to express and regulate emotions
Early elementary (6–9) years	Increased self-reflection; recognition that emotions stem from internal beliefs as well as external situations; simplistic belief in one emotion per situation; reliance on changing the situation or shifting attention to modify emotions
Late elementary (10–12) years	Increased understanding of the complexity of emotional responses; more sophisticated knowledge of cultural/situational norms for expressing emotions; enhanced ability to withhold/hide emotions; emerging ability to reappraise the situation and solve problems

lag in their development of emotional regulation because of poor parenting practices: Their parents are either overly controlling, unpredictable in their emotional responses, or unresponsive. Each of these parenting styles may contribute to a child's sense of insecurity and a limited sense of control over the environment. This diminished sense of control may leave children more vulnerable to anxiety when faced with stressful, novel, or unexpected events (Barlow, 2000). Furthermore, children of parents with more aggressive and coercive parenting styles are more likely to display excessive anger and aggression (Patterson, 2002). In another domain, children's varying levels of language competence (i.e., their ability to label emotions, talk about their feelings, and use self-talk strategies) can also result in a range of emotional control capabilities. Finally, the cultural or social context that children encounter will influence the range and intensity of emotional regulation. For example, some parents, teachers, and peer groups have a greater tolerance for and encourage a broader range and intensity of emotional expression, while others impose restraints on the expression of emotions at home or at school.

Although many students may have occasional difficulties controlling their emotions especially when they are excessively stressed or fatigued, students who have chronic problems with emotional regulation may be at greater risk of or more likely to have an emotional or behavioral disorder. Difficulties in regulating negative emotions (such as worry or sadness) may indicate the presence of an internalizing disorder (such as anxiety or depression), whereas problems with anger and impulsivity suggest the possibility of an externalizing or behavioral disorder (such as ADHD or oppositional defiant disorder). On the other hand, some children may struggle with symptoms of both internalizing and externalizing disorders. In fact, Marmorstein (2007) discovered that there is a strong association between social phobia and aggression, as well as between overanxious disorder and oppositional defiant disorder. In the same vein, children with ADHD often experience considerable anxiety and may be at greater risk for obsessive–compulsive disorder as well (Hallowell & Ratey, 1994).

Emotional Regulation in the Classroom

In the classroom, the ability to modulate and shift emotions is a critical component of effective and efficient learning. As students develop strategies for monitoring and modifying their emotional responses to the social and academic demands of the classroom, they are better able to attend to instruction, sustain their effort, and work through their frustrations when faced with challenging tasks. They also learn to resolve conflicts with peers, collaborate with others, and adjust their behavior to fit the classroom's "culture" and routines. More specifically, students who are skilled at emotional regulation can avoid emotionally triggering situations when needed, ignore critical or hurtful comments from others, focus their attention on the material rather than their inner feelings, use self-talk effectively to encourage themselves when anxious or discouraged, ask for help when needed, and express their feelings in socially acceptable ways. Given this skill set, these students can solve problems more creatively (sustaining their interest and motivation); work more efficiently (without the distraction/burden of strong emotions); and manage the multidimensional demands of advocating for themselves, meeting teacher expectations, and working collaboratively with peers (by keeping their emotions "in check").

However, even students with highly developed emotional control may at times have difficulty when they are faced with an overwhelming academic load or an emotionally laden situation at home (e.g., an abusive home, a chronically sick or dying parent, parental alcoholism or other substance abuse, an impending or recent divorce) or at school (e.g., bullying, rejection, academic failure). Therefore, it is essential that teachers understand how to help all students, and especially those who are struggling, to improve their strategies for regulating their emotions.

HOW CAN WE HELP STUDENTS TO DEVELOP STRATEGIES FOR SELF-REGULATING THEIR EMOTIONS?

Implementing a Formal Emotion-Based Curriculum

Many systemwide programs with the goal of preventing social-emotional difficulties among students have been developed, implemented, and evaluated across the United States. Studies have shown that these social-emotional education programs have resulted in better impulse control, improved problem-solving and conflict resolution skills, decreased aggression and depression, and higher standardized achievement scores (Greenberg, Kusche, Cook, & Quamma, 1995; Hawkins & Catalano, 1992). In fact, "programs that improve students' social and emotional competencies play "a critical role in improving children's academic performance and lifelong learning" (Zins, Bloodworth, Weissberg, & Walberg, 2004, p. 3). Moreover, such programs "foster the development of emotional self-regulation, persistance, cooperation, and goal setting in the classroom and beyond" (Zins, Weissberg, Wang, & Walberg, 2004).

One exemplary program that has been effective in the New England area is the Open Circle curriculum (*www.open-circle.org*), which was designed for kindergarten through fifth grade. This curriculum consists of 35 basic lessons for each grade level, which are presented in a preestablished developmental sequence from kindergarten through fifth grade. The program is designed to provide a forum for open, nonjudgmental discussion of social-emotional issues and to teach specific social-emotional skills within an "open-circle" format. Some of the topics common to all grade levels include listening, cooperating, understanding others' feelings, expressing feelings appropriately, responding to difficult behaviors, and problem solving. Individual lesson plans are tailored to 30-minute discussions. Teachers are encouraged to present two lessons per week and to reinforce the concepts and specific skills throughout the year. A newsletter for parents is also provided so that the lessons can be further discussed and reinforced at home.

In-house evaluation studies (Black, 1995; Timko, 1998), as well as an experimental study (Hennessey, 2007), have documented the program's effectiveness in improving students' social-emotional competence—including an increase in cooperation during academic tasks, a decrease in problematic classroom behaviors, and a decline in peer-related conflicts. When compared to controls, fourth-grade students in both urban and suburban schools made significant gains in their social skills (as rated by their teachers) during the course of a 1-year exposure to the Open Circle curriculum (Siegle, Lange, & Macklem, 1997). In another study, middle school students who had participated in at least 2 years of the Open Circle program in elementary school had better social skills and a higher level of psychosocial adjustment than peers who had little or no exposure to the program (Taylor, Liang, Tracy, Williams, & Seigle, 2002). In general, teachers who have implemented this curriculum in their classrooms have reported that the program has improved student behavior, fostered an acceptance of individual differences, and helped to create a caring classroom environment (Koteff & Seigle, 2006).

Providing Explicit Instruction for Specific Emotional Regulation Skills

Even if teachers are working in schools that have no explicit social-emotional learning program, they have multiple opportunities to make a significant impact on children's emotional development. On a macro level, teachers can play an important role in supporting skill development by providing appropriate modeling (e.g., explicitly sharing their emotions and ways to manage them), strengthening awareness and acceptance of emotions (e.g., empathic listening and reflecting of students' feelings), sharing relevant information that might ease students' distress (e.g., "The highest score on this test was a 75"), and coaching students through difficult situations (e.g., "Why don't you take a break, then try using the strategy we discussed yesterday when tackling that problem?"). At the elementary level, and even at the middle school level, teachers can effectively prompt the kind of emotional control that is desired in the classroom by using verbal as well as visual reminders. Posters and cue cards that explicitly remind students to think through their actions before impulsively responding can help to guide and reinforce student behavior.

Practicing impulse control and other emotional regulation skills is critical for learning. For example, when rules are established in a classroom, they can be first modeled by the teacher, practiced by the class as a whole, and then reinforced by having students role-play situations in which the rules play an important part. If the rule is to refrain from criticizing others' ideas or calling each other names, a teacher might first discuss the negative behavior and its impact on others, demonstrate the desired behavior accompanied by encouraging self-talk, and then have the class practice in pairs or small groups. If the rule is to ask appropriately for help, students can be taught the steps presented in Figure 8.3.

If you think you need help with your work:

1. *Think for yourself:*

   - Have I ever done this before?
   - What do I already know about this topic or task?
   - What can I try to get started?
   - What can I do if I get stuck?

2. *Ask a friend for help.*

3. *If you still need help, then come see me.*

FIGURE 8.3. Steps in asking for help.

Impulse Control

One particularly effective impulse control strategy that has been widely used in clinical and classroom settings, and has empirical support, is the *turtle technique*. This intervention is a cognitive-behavioral strategy that was first developed to teach adults anger management skills and then was adapted for school-age children (Robin, Schneider, & Dolnick, 1976; Schneider, 1974). The turtle technique has been reported to be especially effective in reducing the frequency of aggressive behaviors when taught to aggressive and impulsive children (Robin et al., 1976). To implement this strategy, children are taught four basic steps (see Figure 8.4):

1. Recognize when you are angry (i.e., know the physical signs of anger, such as a clenched jaw, feeling hot in the face, etc.) or otherwise emotionally out of control.
2. Stop and think.
3. Go into your "shell" like a turtle, take three deep breaths, and think calming thoughts.
4. Come out of your shell when you are calm, and think of a solution to the problem.

Other evidence-based cognitive-behavioral interventions for children who struggle with anger management problems, impulsivity, and/or ADHD in the classroom have generally focused on teaching children to be more aware of their attention, emotional state, and behavioral responses, and/or helping them to learn specific self-control strategies or problem-solving steps. For example, Barkley, Copeland, and Sivage (1980) found that the use of taped auditory signals was effective in reducing off-task behavior for children with ADHD. Videotaping both positive and negative responses to anger-provoking situations proved to be effective for some individuals (Booth & Fairbank, 1983). Problem-solving approaches

Step 1. Recognize your feeling.

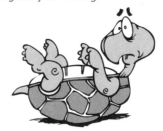

Step 2. Stop and think.

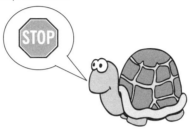

Step 3. Go into your shell and take three deep breaths.

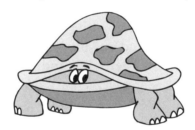

Step 4. Come out of your shell and think of a solution.

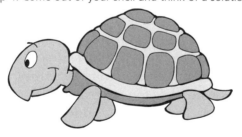

FIGURE 8.4. The turtle technique.

to teaching better self-control have also been shown to be moderately effective in the short run, but less effective over long periods of time (Barkley et al., 1980). For instance, Kendall and Zupan (1981) discovered that their Stop and Think program, a 12-session problem-solving intervention for problem children in grades 3–5, produced significant improvements in self-control among their experimental groups when compared to controls immediately following the treatment; however, at the 2-month follow-up, there were no significant differences among the children in the study. On the other hand, these intervention strategies and problem-solving approaches would probably be more effective if they were taught within the classroom setting, where the emotional triggers and problem situations are more likely to occur. In addition, if children were frequently reminded of the problem-solving steps, prompted to use them in certain situations, and frequently reinforced for doing so, then they would be more likely to internalize the self-control strategies and be able to access them when needed.

Transitions

Although many challenging or emotionally laden situations can derail a student's emotional state, among the most common triggers for emotional upsets at the elementary and middle school levels are *transitions* during the school day. Therefore, teachers can be most helpful to students by proactively planning activities that target emotional regulation at the beginning and end of the day, as well as during other key transition times. Many elementary teachers have found that implementing a "morning meeting" is a time to introduce emotional learning concepts and to encourage discussion of related issues and problems that students may be experiencing. Morning meeting activities often start with a fun greeting, provide opportunities for children to express their opinions or feelings about an activity or topic, and prepare students for the activities of the day. Many creative suggestions for morning meeting activities are available through the *Responsive Classroom Newsletter*, which is published online (*www.responsiveclassroom.org*).

   In addition, transitions between classroom activities/classes, or other breaks in the day, often challenge students to wait patiently and shift their activity level and frame of mind. When teachers explicitly address these issues in the classroom, they are much more successful in helping all students improve their impulse control and other aspects of emotional regulation. For example, if teachers want their students to be able to wait quietly and peacefully in the hallway for the next class, in the classroom for the next lesson, or in the cafeteria line for lunch, then teachers can explicitly teach them a variety of techniques and fun activities to facilitate their ability to wait. Some creative games and activities that can especially help with this issue are presented by Kwane-Ross (2003). Some ideas include having students brainstorm activities they can do while waiting and posting them on a bulletin board; teaching students a number of activities, such as hand-clapping rhymes,

"Rock, Paper, Scissors," "Simon Says," and string games; and reminding students that they can read a book, draw, or practice skills (such as learning new vocabulary, spelling words, or math facts). Kwane-Ross (2003) emphasizes the importance of explicitly discussing the concept of waiting, involving students in generating ideas, modeling the strategies, practicing the wait activities in class, and cueing the students to use these strategies on a consistent basis. Some ideas for activities that could help students learn to wait are presented in Figure 8.5.

Teaching students how to pace themselves appropriately during transitions is another way to maintain an emotionally calm, less stressful classroom environment. One seasoned teacher and consultant has described her method for helping her students manage transitions in the classroom by using a metacognitive strategy (Valentine, 2007, p. 12).

> My observations told me I couldn't assume students knew how to best use the time between the warning and the beginning of cleanup. So I set up a table as if I were in the middle of a project and role-played what I might do after hearing I had five minutes before cleanup. I thought out loud about my stopping place, how I'd organize my cleanup, and how long I estimated things would take. I asked the children to help me problem solve. Then I had volunteers role-play how they would handle the same situation, showing there could be more than one approach.

Waiting Task	Possible Activities
Waiting in line	Play a hand game with a friend.
	Imagine that you're in a favorite place or are your favorite character.
	Practice your spelling words for the week.
	Play a guessing game with a friend, such as "20 Questions," "I Spy," or "Geography."
	Play a string game with a partner.
	Start a round of "Telephone."
Waiting at your desk for the next activity	Read a book.
	Draw a picture.
	Play solitaire.
	Work on a crossword puzzle or word search.
	Write a poem or short story.
	Practice spelling words or math facts.
	Make a card for a good friend or family member.
Waiting in a lunch line	Decide what you want for lunch.
	Look for friends to sit with.
	Think about what you want to do during recess or free block.
	Use your imagination to create an idea for a short story, poem, movie, or play.
	Play a guessing game with a friend.

FIGURE 8.5. Waiting activities.

For a while, we practiced in "real life" situations by stopping after the five-minute warning and asking a few students to share their wrapping-up plans. Then we'd proceed, and they'd try out their plans. After cleanup, they'd report on what worked, what didn't, and what they might do differently next time.

Providing Appropriate Academic Supports to Decrease Emotional Triggers

Accommodations

Facing an overwhelming or challenging academic task is another stressful situation for many students, especially those with learning or attention difficulties. They may be easily frustrated, overcome by anxiety, or so discouraged that they avoid the assignment altogether. In fact, the phrase "Your homework assignment is on the board" may send some students into a panic as they conjure up images of endless hours of tedious worksheets. They may be flooded by overwhelming feelings of confusion and frustration as they try to recall how to finish their math homework, or imagine the pressure and stress associated with evenings that include no "down time" for e-mailing or texting friends, relaxing with a book, or playing a game. Some children are exhausted by the academic and social demands of the school day and have had years of experience struggling to complete assignments within a reasonable time frame. Teachers can effectively assist such students in coping with academic challenges by ensuring that they have the necessary supports and accommodations in place. Teachers can also ensure that assignments are designed appropriately, so that students can rely on their strengths and be rewarded for their efforts. In addition, students can be specifically taught how to use self-talk and self-reflection strategies to help them cope with the pressures of their schoolwork.

When students are given the accommodations and extra help that they need on a consistent basis, their stress levels can become much more manageable. However, some teachers feel uncomfortable with providing accommodations all the time. Perhaps they want to challenge students occasionally or test the continued need for an accommodation. Consider Jack, for example, who depended on using a calculator or math fact chart to complete his fifth-grade in-class math assignments and tests. Sporadically, his teacher would decide that "no calculators" were allowed to be used that day. This decision would send Jack into a panic not only for that day but for many mornings, as he anxiously wondered whether his teacher would make the same decision again. Similarly, Annie, a high school sophomore with poor executive function skills, depended on extended deadlines for major written assignments in order to manage her workload. If it was unclear to her whether she could have an extension in a particular class, Annie would often become paralyzed with anxiety and sometimes would end up with a migraine, both of which further impaired her ability to complete her assignments. Given the fact that anxiety and executive function processes are inversely related—that is, one cannot efficiently deploy these processes and be highly anxious at the same time—students need the safety and security of knowing that they can consistently rely on their needed accommodations in order for them to perform at their best.

Rubrics

Sometimes anxiety and confusion among students can be reduced when teachers offer clear assignments that are broken down into manageable steps, and when they provide opportunities for students to choose the topic, modality, or format of the finished product (Stein & Krishnan, 2007). Studies of achievement and motivation have identified students' choice, control, and confidence in their ability to accomplish tasks as important factors that enhance their motivation and performance (Deci & Ryan, 1985; Dweck, 2006; Vansteenkiste, Simons, Lens, Sheldon, & Deci, 2004). Teachers who know their students' strengths and abilities can more effectively plan assignments that will enhance students' motivation and success while minimizing their stress level. Students' ownership of their work, and hence their motivation, can be improved by offering a variety of options with respect to assignments and by providing very explicit expectations and criteria for the quality of work desired. When students have an opportunity to choose the format of their work and know how to meet the teacher's expectations for an assignment, they will probably be more motivated to perform at a higher level.

Self-Talk and Self-Reflection Strategies

Another effective way that teachers can improve students' ability to master the emotional aspects of learning within the classroom is to explicitly teach and reinforce the use of self-talk and self-reflection strategies. A research-based model for embedding self-talk strategies into the classroom curriculum has been described by Graham, Harris, and Olinghouse (2007a). They have developed and implemented a strategic approach to writing that incorporates a self-regulation component. In their program, students are taught effective strategies for writing (e.g., POW: Put down your ideas, Organize them, and Write/write more), as well as specific ways to use self-talk to manage their anxiety, self-doubt, and frustration while composing an essay. Specifically, students are guided to create a list of self-statements to address any emotional responses that might impede their progress, as well as to reinforce the effort and strategy use that they are expending to complete the assignment. As with any effective instructional program, the self-regulation strategies are first modeled by the teacher multiple times as he or she works through planning and writing an essay; are then practiced in small groups with teacher support; and are finally implemented individually with prompts (cue cards or teacher reminders) that are faded over time.

HOW CAN WE TAKE A PROACTIVE APPROACH
TO HELPING STUDENTS WITH THEIR EMOTIONS?

A proactive approach to addressing emotional regulation in the classroom involves three critical components: (1) knowing the students, (2) understanding what kinds of triggers may upset each student, and (3) developing an individualized prevention and intervention plan for the most vulnerable students.

Knowing the Students

At the beginning of each academic year, teachers can get to know their students by scheduling brief conferences with each individual to review his or her strengths, challenges, interests, goals, and expectations for the class. By discussing each student's learning style and his or her academic goals, teachers can assess what kinds of assignments would be most appropriate and anticipate what kinds of academic tasks might be most frustrating. In this way, teachers can identify those students who are most vulnerable to becoming overwhelmed, easily frustrated, or emotionally distraught. Teachers will need to pay particular attention to those students who have a known diagnosis (ADHD, a nonverbal learning disorder, an anxiety disorder, a bipolar disorder, obsessive–compulsive disorder, an autism spectrum disorder, a seizure disorder) or have experienced significant trauma (living in an orphanage, deaths, accidents, violence, parental depression, or parental substance abuse). In addition, teachers might notice which students are most reluctant to participate in classroom discussions, are slow in completing their work, ask for help frequently, give up easily when facing challenges, and have difficulty with transitions and adapting to change.

Understanding Each Student's Triggers

Although understanding each student's triggers may seem like an overwhelming endeavor, it is necessary to identify those tasks and situations that are most likely to create distress, in order to facilitate a safe and positive learning environment. For example, a student who has difficulty working in a group should be given a chance to work alone or with a carefully selected partner. If test taking is a common trigger for anxiety or distress, then problem solving with the student before a test to develop a plan will be an important step in alleviating the anxiety. For some students, a change in routine or an unexpected challenge could set off a "false-alarm" panic-stricken reaction. For example, if a student is reliant on having extra time for tests, being asked to do "fast math" on the computer may trigger an intense emotional reaction. This bout of anxiety may then create a vicious cycle of anticipatory anxiety, test anxiety, poor performance, and eventual shutdown. By talking with parents and previous teachers, carefully observing students for signs

Date/time	Situation	Trigger	Emotional response
Monday 10:00	Math test	Forgot calculator	Put head on desk, didn't start test
Tuesday 2:00	Group project	Partner shot down idea	Angry outburst, left room
Wednesday 3:00	Wrap-up of school day	Homework announced	Panic-stricken face, groans, complaints
Thursday 9:00	Substitute teacher	Teacher changed morning routine	Refused to follow instructions, started doodling
Friday 11:00	Learning center	Accused of writing in textbook	Loud denial, agitation, crying
Friday 1:00	Cafeteria	Peer moved as she sat down at table	Walked out of cafeteria, head down, without eating

FIGURE 8.6. Record of emotional triggers for a student.

of emotional distress, and charting each episode of emotional overload, teachers can identify the most common triggers. An example of a list of triggers that upset one student is provided in Figure 8.6.

If there are more than one or two students in a class who are having significant difficulty regulating their emotions and executive function processes, then assistance from the special education team and/or guidance department to observe and record problematic incidents occurring in the classroom or on the school grounds may be necessary.

Planning Ahead

Once the common triggers have been identified for the most vulnerable students, then an individualized plan of prevention and intervention can be developed for each student.

Prevention

Every prevention plan will need to incorporate these components:

- Identify ways to avoid known triggers as much as possible.
- Develop a plan with the student for handling unavoidable triggers.

- Inform all teachers, helpers, substitutes, and aides of the student's specific triggers.
- Embed self-regulation strategies into lesson plans (e.g., demonstrate positive self-talk, discuss what to do if the student gets stuck, normalize mistakes as part of the learning process, explain a variety of ways to approach a new task).
- Ensure that necessary accommodations are in place at all times.
- Make sure that the student understands assignments and due dates.
- Help the student get started before frustration sets in: Model the task or break it down into smaller steps.
- Offer an alternative assignment, test format, or second chance if the student is having a "bad day."
- Provide flexible due dates as needed (within reason—i.e., 1 or 2 extra days).
- Warn the student of upcoming changes, transitions, new units, challenges, or requests for participation.
- Positively reinforce successful and improved attempts at self-regulation.
- Provide explicit guidelines and study tips; talk through assignments; and provide models for homework, novel tasks, projects, and upcoming tests.

Intervention

In order for an intervention plan to be effective, the following guidelines may be helpful:

- Intervene quickly at the first signs of distress.
- Have a written plan for intervention accessible to all staff members and the student.
- Have a backup support person a teacher or other staff member can call if the situation becomes unmanageable.
- When a student is upset, listen empathically first, and then reflect back what the student has said.
- Keep the conversation calm and friendly; avoid judgment, anger, blame, and impatience at all costs.
- Be respectful and supportive, maintaining a collaborative frame of mind: "let's figure out what's wrong and see if we can find a solution together."
- Offer choices (e.g., destressing, going to a safe place, taking a test in a quiet room, working alone).

Teachers must keep in mind that the main goal is to diminish the level of distress and to reengage the executive function system (controlled by the brain's frontal lobes). Little learning or production will occur until both tasks are accomplished. (See "Calming the Emotional Brain" and "Firing Up the Frontal Lobes," below, for specific strategies.)

HOW CAN TEACHERS BE EFFECTIVE
WHEN STUDENTS BECOME EMOTIONALLY DISTRAUGHT?

When teachers are faced with emotionally laden or highly stressful situations in the classroom, they have multiple opportunities to intervene in an effective way. As illustrated by Gross and Thompson's (2007) model of emotional regulation, an intervention can be targeted at each of the steps in the development of an emotional response (see Figure 8.7). That is, when a vulnerable student is facing a potentially stressful task or interaction, a teacher can decide to intervene by changing or eliminating the situation, directing the student to modify his or her attentional focus, suggesting an alternative interpretation of the situation, or guiding the student to express his or her feelings appropriately.

In some cases, teachers may choose to intervene at the situational level so that a student is less likely to react in a negative or maladaptive way. For example, if a student becomes highly anxious and dysfunctional when given "mad minute" math assessments, a teacher may choose to eliminate this kind of assessment for this individual. For another student with a similar issue, a teacher may choose to modify the test so that it covers only those facts that the student has mastered.

A teacher may also intervene at the attentional level by either distracting a student who is overly upset about a situation or prompting the student to focus more intently on a particular aspect of his or her reaction. If a student is ruminating about his or her poor performance on a test and getting increasingly upset, a teacher may choose to distract the student by asking about an upcoming sports event in which he or she is participating. Or the teacher may try to focus the student's attention on the test questions that were answered correctly.

Alternatively, a teacher can intervene at the stage of cognitive appraisal of the situation. That is, the teacher can help the student modify or reframe his or her assessment of the situation. If a student is experiencing "writer's block" and becoming extremely frustrated, a teacher might point out that all skilled writers have writer's block on occasion, and then congratulate the student on "joining the ranks" of the very best authors. Or the teacher might ask the student what he or

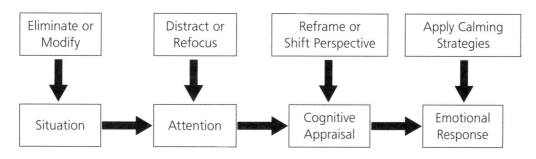

FIGURE 8.7. A model of intervention. Based on Gross and Thompson (2007).

she might say to a friend who was experiencing a similar paralysis. By helping the student shift his or her perspective and role (from those of a writer to those of a friend), the teacher can help him or her to reframe the situation and thus to gain more effective emotional control.

Finally, if all else fails, or the opportunity to intervene earlier has passed, teachers can help students modulate their emotional responses. For instance, a student who is already very angry at a peer for teasing him or her can be reminded of the rules ("Use your words, not your fists") and coached to take a walk, count to 10, use an "I" statement, or express his or her feelings in a calm voice. Moreover, teachers can significantly influence their students' level of distress and emotion-driven behavior by encouraging and reinforcing appropriate emotional responses (e.g., "I'm so impressed by the way you handled that difficult essay question. You stayed calm and kept working until you were finished"). The power of positive reinforcement is often underestimated by teachers, but it has repeatedly been shown to be an important component of highly effective classrooms (Reynolds & Teddlie, 1999).

In the next section, we offer some general suggestions for helping students deal with anxiety—an emotion that can have a particularly devastating effect on their efforts to attain academic success.

WHAT ARE SOME GENERAL STRATEGIES FOR HELPING ANXIOUS STUDENTS TO CALM THEMSELVES?

Labeling and Normalizing Anxiety

Almost everyone feels anxious at times. In fact, it is the human body's natural reaction to stress. When our minds perceive a threat, our bodies becomes prepared to fight, flee, or freeze in order to protect ourselves from danger. Unfortunately, sometimes our brains perceive a situation as dangerous when it really is not. In such cases, the anxiety works against us, shutting down the thinking parts of our brains when we may need our cognitive functioning to be at our best. The goal is to maintain a useful level of anxiety and not let it take charge.

Students also need to know the typical course for anxiety. Teachers can explain that anxiety will generally be short-lived. It will increase gradually, reach a peak, and then diminish over time. Teachers can compare the experience of having an anxiety reaction to the experience of riding a wave or riding a bicycle up and down a hill (see Figure 8.8). In other words, anxiety will often build when a difficult situation arises, but if a student can sit with the feeling and continue doing the task, the anxiety will diminish and the student will feel relief.

To help students experience the ups and downs of their anxiety, it's helpful to have them map it out during a day. Teachers can suggest that students rate their level of anxiety from 1 ("little or no anxiety") to 10 ("out of control—panic city!").

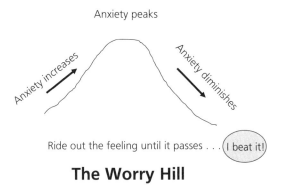

The Worry Hill

FIGURE 8.8. The "worry hill." Adapted from Wagner (2005). Copyright 2005 by Lighthouse Press, Inc. Adapted by permission. Worry Hill is a registered trademark of Lighthouse Press, Inc.

Figure 8.9 is Mark's anxiety chart, which shows that each of the peaks occurred during a math lesson or homework time.

Reminding Students of Their Past Successes

Another clinically useful strategy is to remind students of their past successes (see Figure 8.10) and/or help them to imagine future successes when they confront a difficult situation or perform an especially challenging task. Visualizing the situation and their desired response is likely to enhance their confidence and their ability to handle the anxiety-provoking endeavor.

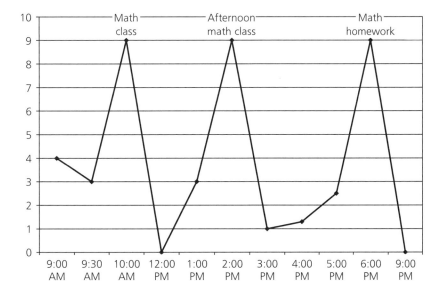

FIGURE 8.9. Chart of a student's anxiety level.

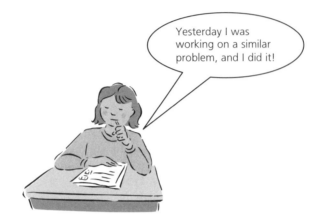

FIGURE 8.10. Reminders of past successes.

Teaching Effective Self-Talk Strategies

As described previously, teachers have many opportunities to model and teach positive self-talk strategies that will help students cope with stressful situations. It may be important for teachers to verbalize self-statements first, encourage students to generate their own, and then instruct them to write them down. Students will then have to be reminded and cued to use their self-talk when they are facing an emotionally or academically challenging task. Again, for example, consider Mark, who had struggled with math anxiety for a long time. As soon as math class began and he was asked to work on problems independently, his mind immediately shifted into negative thinking (e.g., "I can't do it. I'll probably get stuck. I won't finish. It'll take forever!"). With coaching and practice, however, Mark was able to learn how to modify his thinking so that he could tackle his math assignments without excessive anxiety. Some of the more positive self-statements he generated are listed in Figure 8.11.

Calming the Emotional Brain

All students will experience times in their school careers when their anxiety (or some other emotion) overwhelms them and interferes with their performance in the classroom or elsewhere. Therefore, it is important for all students to learn some basic skills in coping with stressful situations. At the elementary school level, teachers might choose to allocate some time each week (or even daily) to learn and practice calming techniques. Others may choose to have a guidance counselor or psychologist present a series of workshops or meetings to discuss these coping strategies. At the middle school and high school level, instruction can take place during guidance groups, health/wellness classes, or homeroom periods. Class-room teachers can then be mindful of these coping methods and cue their students to use them as needed.

> 1. I've tried these kinds of problems before. I can do them again.
>
> 2. I can do the easy ones first and then ease into the more difficult ones.
>
> 3. If I get stuck, I can ask for help.
>
> 4. If I make a mistake, it'll be OK.

FIGURE 8.11. Examples of a student's Positive self-talk.

Destressing

To help an anxious student destress, a teacher can say something like this:

"I can see that you are really worried/upset about this [test or other situation]. Let's see if you feel better if we take a walk down the hall, get a drink, relax in our cozy corner, and talk about what you're so worried about, or use our bodies to let go of the stress. We can do push-ups against a wall, press our feet into the floor, or first go stiff like a robot and then go limp like a beanbag."

Using a Real or Imagined Safe Place

Teachers can help all of their students to identify a real or imagined place where they feel perfectly calm, safe, secure, and peaceful. A calm feeling is more easily accessed if the place is a real one—perhaps a place students have been on vacation; a cozy place in their room or home; or a place where they feel most successful, such as the dancing studio, music school, stage, or basketball court. If students cannot identify a safe place, then they can imagine one (see Figure 8.12). Students should close their eyes and bring up a detailed image of the safe place, noticing with all of their senses what the place looks, feels, smells, and sounds, and (if appropriate) tastes like. When the image is really strong, they can "mark" this place on their bodies (by squeezing tightly the area just above a knee, or a wrist, or the upper knuckle of a thumb or pinky) so they can easily come back to it when they need it (Shapiro, 1995).

Surfing the "Worry Wave"

Students can be taught that worry and anxiety are normal and that they come and go like a wave in the ocean. The trick is to ride the "worry wave" through to the end until it comes to shore, as if they were riding a surfboard, rather than getting swallowed up by it and knocked off the surfboard. One way of learning to ride the worry wave out is for them to take several deep breaths and reassure themselves

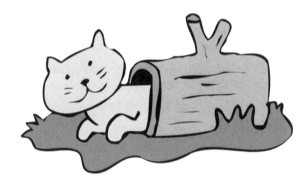

FIGURE 8.12. Relaxing image of a safe place.

with encouraging self-talk: "This is just a worry wave. I can ride it out and stay on top. It will pass very soon. In the meantime, I can take deep breaths or imagine a peaceful, safe place I'd like to be. (This strategy is based on Wagner, 2005; see Figure 8.9).

Mindfulness Meditation

Students can be taught to focus their attention on their breathing. They can be encouraged to place their hands on their stomachs, then their rib cages, and finally their chests, to feel their breath. They can be told to imagine that there is a balloon in their bellies inflating and deflating as they breathe in peacefulness and breathe out tension/stress. Students can be encouraged to let their thoughts gently float in, to notice them, and then to let them float out (like a leaf on the surface of the water, a sailboat crossing a lake, a bird gliding in the sky, or a hot air balloon slowly rising). Then they can return to focusing on their breath.

Focusing: Clearing a Space

Students can be taught to relax and to distance themselves from their feelings and stresses by clearing an inner space (see, e.g., Gendlin, 1981). The instructions can be given as follows:

> "Close your eyes and take a few deep breaths as you settle into your chair in a comfortable position. Notice how your feet feel on the floor, your body feels in the chair, your hands feel on your lap. . . . Focus your attention inside in the center of your body . . notice what's there. . . . Then you might ask yourself, 'What's between how you feel now and feeling really good?' or 'What's getting in the way of your feeling really good right now?' Let the answers come from your body. . . . As you become aware of any tensions, feelings, or stresses, imagine wrapping them up in a package and putting them outside of your body at just the right distance. . . . Take each feeling or worry or problem, and

wrap it up and put it outside of you, knowing you can come back to any of these feelings or concerns later if you want to. . . . Now see if there's any background feeling/tension/stress that you may be carrying around with you, and wrap that up and put it aside. Check your body from head to toe, and make sure you've wrapped up every bit of worry or stress. Now that you've cleared a space for yourself inside, notice how you feel and spend a moment enjoying you as you are right now . . . just being, not having to do anything. [After a minute or so] Then gently come back to the room."

If there is time, the students can then draw or write down what their worries or concerns were, and what it was like after they cleared a space.

Firing Up the Frontal Lobes

When students are already in a panic-stricken state or shut-down mode, they will need to be guided through a process of lowering their level of emotional arousal and shifting their focus in order to reengage the executive function system—a process that can be referred to as "firing up the frontal lobes" (see Figure 8.13). Therapists have developed many techniques that can help highly stressed individuals to set aside their emotions, to think more clearly, and to reconnect with the people around them (Levine & Kline, 2006; Ogden, Minton, & Pain, 2006).

Grounding Students in the Moment

Students can be asked what they are feeling in the moment. In other words, teachers can ask them to describe their state of mind, to observe what sensations they feel in their bodies, and to notice how their feelings change.

Widening the Focus/Perspective

Students can be directed to look around the room, to take in the "big picture," to look at a teacher, or to read the situation.

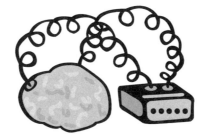

FIGURE 8.13. Firing up the frontal lobes.

Asking a Question with Curiosity

Some useful questions include "What's the crux of this issue?", "What is the worst part of this situation?", and "What image or word captures all of this?"

Changing Viewpoint

Teachers might encourage students to take the perspective of a good friend or a family member: "What would your best friend say/do in this situation?" or "What would you tell your best friend or little brother/sister to do in this situation?"

Expanding the Time Frame

Helping students to get some distance from the upsetting circumstances can diminish the intensity of their feelings. Asking questions about the past or future can redirect the students' focus and change their emotional response. For example, teachers can ask:

- "Have you ever felt like this before?"
- "What happened then?"
- "What was the outcome?"
- "What's a first step you could take now that would help?"

By enabling students to refocus their attention, become more aware of their surroundings, and begin to reflect on their experience, teachers can help students to calm down sufficiently that they can return to the academic task that needs to be addressed. Once their level of arousal has returned to an optimal level, students can utilize their cognitive abilities and executive function skills to tackle the problem at hand.

For those students who are particularly difficult to calm down, teachers may need to develop a backup plan that involves other professionals. If a student is struggling without success to regain control over his or her emotions, then a teacher will need to call upon a guidance counselor, nurse, psychologist, or administrator to intervene in an appropriate manner.

Helping Students Evaluate the Results of Their Efforts

Teachers can help their students to assess their own emotional and behavioral responses to difficult encounters and the effectiveness of their plans. Some of the important questions that students can be encouraged to ask include the following:

- "Did I get the outcome I wanted?"
- "Was I less anxious than I thought I would be?"

- "How did others respond?"
- "What did I do that was most helpful?"
- "What could I do differently next time?"

Finally, teachers should encourage their students to reward themselves for working hard and trying to manage their anxiety while being productive. In this way, students will learn to acknowledge their own successes and to reflect on the process of applying self-regulation strategies. Their efforts can be then be self-rewarded (by giving themselves praise or a concrete reward), or can be reinforced by a special privilege, activity, or treat provided by the teacher. Some useful questions to guide students' thinking about their ability to use their coping skills are as follows:

- "Did I face my fears?"
- "Did I use effective self-talk or other coping skills?"
- "Did I complete the task or endure the situation?"
- "What can I say and do to celebrate?"

CONCLUSION

As teachers reflect on ways that they can improve executive function processes among their students, it is important that they consult with school counselors or school psychologists who can help them to incorporate preventive and responsive strategies for fostering the development of effective emotional regulation. Research studies have shown that with well-developed self-regulation skills, students can modulate their levels of energy, motivation, frustration tolerance, and anxiety so that they can more readily access their cognitive resources (attention, memory, problem solving, language, planning, organization, and self-monitoring) and direct these toward new learning and stronger academic performance. Teachers have many opportunities to assist their students in acquiring and refinding emotional regulation skills. They can choose to implement a formal social-emotional learning program in their classrooms; incorporate components of emotional intelligence into their regular subject-oriented lesson plans; develop specific behavioral support plans for emotionally vulnerable students; or focus on helping students to negotiate particularly challenging academic tasks, such as taking a final exam or writing a research paper. Ideally, the various ideas and strategies presented in this chapter will provide a foundation as well as a springboard for improving students' emotional functioning in the classroom.

PART III

CASE STUDIES

Addressing Executive Function Weaknesses across the Grades

LENA HANNUS-SUKSI, LAURA SALES POLLICA, WENDY STACEY, MELISSA J. FELLER, and JASON BENDEZU

Chris, 11-Year-Old Fifth Grader

Executive Function Weaknesses That Affect Organizing, Prioritizing, Planning, Shifting

BACKGROUND

Chris is an 11-year-old fifth grader. His parents and teachers describe him as an enthusiastic and energetic young boy who is sociable and generally well liked by his peers. He also enjoys karate and swimming. Chris has always struggled in the classroom. Last year he was referred for a neurospsychological and educational evaluation, but the results indicated that he did not meet the criteria for the diagnosis of a learning disability or ADHD. According to reports from Chris's teachers, his performance has never matched his potential. His parents have always had a difficult time getting him to start assignments and complete his homework on time. Similarly, he has often completed long-term projects at the last minute or turned them in late. Chris often forgets to bring his books to school and appears disheveled when entering the classroom; when he does have his materials with him, they are usually scattered in his backpack. His teacher reports that Chris often spends more time looking for his assignments than actually working on them. He also struggles to prioritize information in reading comprehension assignments. He generally responds correctly to questions about specific details, but has difficulty with questions relating to the main ideas and major themes. His writing is often a stream of thoughts without a definitive beginning or conclusive ending. Despite his parents' best efforts, Chris put off studying for his most recent vocabulary test and received a failing grade.

During the past year, Chris's parents have hired an educational therapist to help Chris with his reading and writing. The therapist found at first that Chris had difficulty remembering and applying strategies for individual assignments. In addition, Chris was initially reluctant to try out some of the new strategies she suggested.

RECOMMENDATIONS

A year later, a collaborative effort between Chris's teacher and his educational therapist has made a significant difference for Chris. Chris has been using the BOTEC strategy (Brainstorm, Organize, Topic sentence, Evidence, Conclusion; see Chap-

TABLE III.1. Chris, 11-Year-Old Fifth Grader

Executive function weaknesses	Educational difficulties	Recommended strategies	Accommodations
Planning	• Writing is disorganized • Leaves preparation for tests and long-term projects to the last minute	• BOTEC (see Chapter 2) • Weekly calendar with specific goals • Timelines	• Teacher-prompted planning sheets • Daily classroom schedule posted in a central location • Teacher-created class calendar with important due dates/assignments
Organizing	• Struggles to organize information from readings • Does not differentiate main ideas and details • Cluttered workspace • Unprepared for class; lacks materials necessary to complete work	• Triple Note Tote (see Chapters 2 and 4) • Color-coded folders/binders for different classes • Two-pocket homework folder (left: "to-do" side, right: "finished" side) • Backpack with organizers	• Classroom notebook filing system for completed and to-be-completed homework, class work, and notes
Prioritizing	• Spends too much time on small assignments and not enough time on bigger, open-ended projects • Focuses on minor details in his written work, but misses the "big picture"	• Time estimation worksheets • Daily "to-do" lists • Mapping and webbing	• Teacher estimates the time Chris should spend working on assignments • Teacher prioritizes assignments based on their importance • Teacher provides clear expectations and examples
Shifting	• Only sees one way to solve a problem • Reluctant to use strategies and alternative approaches	• Strategy notebook • M & M strategy (see Chapter 6) • Trying alternative plans for the same problem (e.g., Plan A, Plan B) • Venn diagrams (see chapter 6)	• Teacher uses warm-ups at the beginning of classes (e.g., jokes, riddles, multiple-meaning words) to encourage flexible thinking • Teacher incorporates part–whole activities, analogies

ter 2) and mapping out his thoughts on paper, both of which have helped him to plan his written assignments. For long-term projects, he has used planning sheets with his teachers to identify the goal, plan of action, deadline, and anticipated final results. Using a timeline in conjunction with a daily planner has helped Chris to plan his time and follow through on open-ended projects. Color-coding his folders by subject area has also helped Chris stay organized. In the classroom, his teachers have modeled organizational strategies with a notebook filing system for classwork, homework, and notes. When Chris has had trouble gauging how long it will take to complete assignments, he has referred back to his teacher's estimate. Chris has also been using a strategy notebook with sections (e.g., reading, writing, organization) to help him access the appropriate strategies more efficiently. The strategy notebook has served as a reminder of all the strategies he can use to prepare for tests or written assignments. Chris has also added new strategies that he has learned during the year to the strategy notebook. Table III.1 summarizes all of the recommended strategies and accommodations for Chris.

CASE 2

Jenny, 13-Year-Old Seventh Grader
Executive Function Weaknesses That Affect
Working Memory, Organizing, Planning, Prioritizing

BACKGROUND

Jenny is an extremely social seventh grader with above-average verbal reasoning and language abilities. She is an active class participant who does especially well with collaborative and hands-on projects in her classes. However, her academic performance has been inconsistent. Last year Jenny was diagnosed with ADHD and visual–spatial difficulties. Her executive function weaknesses and her inattention have influenced her school performance in several ways. She has struggled with multistep problems in math and has had difficulty keeping track of what she reads. She has also struggled to take notes in class. She has had difficulty remembering important information in science, geography, and history. In addition, Jenny has been highly distractible in class, and her attention has wavered. As a result, she has performed poorly on tests, and her grades have often not reflected her ability or knowledge level. When confronted with assignments that have required her to plan ahead in a step-by-step manner (e.g., multistep projects, research papers), she has had difficulty breaking down tasks into small steps and following the projects through to completion. Because Jenny has found many school situations overwhelming and frustrating, she has often procrastinated with her schoolwork and has preferred spending time with friends instead. Jenny's difficulties with organization have also compromised her ability to keep track of her materials, and she has often lost her handouts and homework. Jenny's parents have acknowledged her struggle with attention and organization, and they recognize the adverse impact this struggle has had on Jenny's school performance.

RECOMMENDATIONS

Through collaboration with her teachers and her tutor, Jenny has learned many useful strategies that have brought greater consistency to her academic performance. For example, she now makes efficient use of mnemonics such as verbal associations, acronyms, and crazy phrases in order to chunk and remember important names, dates, and facts in science, history, and geography. Inventing stories and visualizing also help her to memorize information more effectively. In order to read actively, to better sustain her attention, and to understand what she reads, Jenny has learned to use graphic organizers such as the STAR strategy (see Chapters 2 and 5). This strategy, together with summarizing paragraphs and chapters on Post-it Notes, has helped Jenny to read long texts and write reports. In math, Jenny's tutor has introduced procedure lists (which break procedures down into numbered steps) and acronyms (e.g., RAPS; Read and Rephrase, Art, Plan and Predict, Solve; see Chapter 5 and Appendix 11) to help her more effectively break down and approach math problems that require organizational skills and careful attention to numerous details. After months of practice, Jenny is more confident about using these strategies independently. She also seems more willing to persist with her math. For written assignments, Jenny has been encouraged to use a laptop computer, which she carries with her between school and home. This helps her to organize her assignments and keep track of her work. In addition, she often uses time-planning sheets and makes "to-do" lists to help her organize her time, as well as to prioritize her school tasks versus her social life.

Jenny's strategy use has been encouraged and supported by her teachers. They require Jenny as well as her classmates to complete strategy reflection sheets, which they count toward the grade. In each classroom, there is a display of memory and organizational strategies on a wall, which has helped both Jenny and her classmates with organization and planning. Jenny's teachers also check her homework and her strategy reflection sheets regularly, to monitor effective strategy use. A daily classroom schedule with goals and time limits for each lesson is also on display, to help Jenny and her peers prioritize and make efficient use of their time.

Recently Jenny had a map test in geography that required her to memorize over 70 unfamiliar terms, including countries, cities, landforms, and bodies of water. Together with her tutor, Jenny developed a study plan. She used several memory strategies to prepare for the test, including word associations (to match countries with cities) and acronyms (e.g., CAPP—Cape Horn, Andes Mountains,

Patagonia, Pampas). Jenny was extremely successful and earned 92% on her test! She also received extra credit for completing a strategy reflection sheet in which she described the strategies she had used to study.

Table III.2 summarizes the recommended strategies and accommodations for Jenny.

TABLE III.2. Jenny, 13-Year-Old Seventh Grader

Executive function weaknesses	Educational difficulties	Recommended strategies	Accommodations
Organizing, accessing working memory	• Recalling names, dates, and facts in history, science, and geography • Remembering math facts • Breaking down multistep problems • Organizing information from readings; reading comprehension • Keeping track of information while reading • Taking notes in class • Test taking	• Mnemonics: Associations, acronyms, Crazy Phrases • Visualization • Verbal memory strategies: Rhymes, songs, stories • Procedure lists to keep track of steps • Graphic organizers (e.g., STAR strategy, chapter summary organizer), Post-it Notes • Bypass strategies (e.g., use of a calculator or multiplication charts in math, word banks in science) • Use of an outline to assist with note taking • Access to notes from a classmate or teacher	• Teachers encourage and require use of strategies for homework and class assignments • "Top Ten Strategies" displayed on a strategy board in the classroom • Teachers give extra points for use of strategies on tests and for completion of strategy reflection sheets • Monitoring of progress and strategy use through frequent evaluations and check-ins • Teachers allow use of bypass strategies and extended time for tests
Organizing, planning, prioritizing	• Keeping track of materials • Completing and handing in homework, written assignments, and long-term projects • Being on time to class • Procrastination; balancing school work with extracurricular activities and social life	• Use of laptop for written assignments in school and at home • Keeping belongings in same place (backpack) • Organizational strategies: Calendar, "to-do" lists" mini-goals for long-term projects, assignment notebook, time-planning sheets, study plan	• Teachers allow use of laptop • Teachers provide time each week for students to clean out backpacks and binders • Daily classroom schedule, syllabus, and timelines clearly visible in class • Teachers provide guidelines and strategy tips for completing tasks • Frequent homework and notebook checks

CASE 3

> # Lucy, 15-Year-Old 10th Grader
> *Executive Function Weaknesses That Affect Working Memory, Organizing, Self-Monitoring, Self-Checking*

BACKGROUND

Lucy is a highly motivated 10th grader diagnosed with ADHD and a learning disability, which are reflected in her poor math performance. She has had difficulties retaining math concepts, as well as classroom procedures and instructions. Over the years, she has benefited from multiple exposures to information as well as many opportunities for practice. Because of her difficulties, Lucy has needed individual math support on an after-school basis. When she has put forth the effort, Lucy has been able to learn many math concepts and operations in isolation. However, she has felt overwhelmed when tasks have required her to integrate and apply concepts to more complex problems. Attentional weaknesses have also made it difficult for her to access her knowledge and to self-monitor, so she has always made "careless" mistakes.

RECOMMENDATIONS

Lucy's educational therapy sessions have been geared toward clarifying new content and teaching her strategies for remembering essential information. Lucy has created strategy cards for important formulae and step-by-step math procedures. She has also worked with her educational therapist to develop creative strategies for remembering procedures. In addition, her math teacher has provided her with weekly after-school math review sessions.

Lucy's classroom teacher has also developed activities that help students to understand their learning styles and enhance their metacognitive awareness. For example, she has used strategy reflection sheets with homework and tests to encourage students to self-reflect and apply strategies to their daily work. Lucy's class has also met regularly in small groups to share and discuss the strategies they have used. Lists of metacognitive questions and prompts, as well as procedure lists, have helped Lucy to approach multistep problems systematically and to monitor her work more effectively. For example, the following metacognitive prompts have been helpful in geometry:

1. Which quadrilateral am I working with? Is it a parallelogram? A kite? A rectangle?

2. What do I know about this quadrilateral? Think SAD—Sides, Angles, Diagonals. Check my strategy cards for other characteristics!

3. How do I know which sides or angles are congruent?

During tests, Lucy has also benefited from using personal checklists that she has created with her teacher to find and correct errors that she commonly makes when completing assignments. She has also used her own strategy, "Top Three Hits," to remind her to "(1) work slowly, (2) check as you go, and (3) flag difficult tasks and go back to them later."

Lucy's classroom teacher has emphasized the benefits of strategy use for all her students. On tests, she has permitted all her students to use checklists, strategy cards, and individual strategy notebooks. Table III.3 summarizes the recommended strategies and accommodations for Lucy (and, often, for her peers).

TABLE III.3. Lucy, 15-Year-Old 10th Grader

Executive function weaknesses	Educational difficulties	Recommended strategies	Accommodations
Memorizing, organizing	• Remembering and accessing concepts and procedures in math • Poor performance on tests and quizzes • Note taking in class	• Strategy cards and strategy notebook • Crazy Phrases and acronyms to remember order of operations in math (e.g., BEDMAS; see Chapter 5) • Access to outlines or templates during lessons to scaffold information for note taking	• Teacher allows time for explicit strategy instruction and practice, and integrates strategies into the curriculum • Monthly and yearly strategy goals • Mastery and use of strategies required and encouraged by teacher ("effort" grade, Strategy Reflection Sheets)
Working memory, self-monitoring, self-checking	• Manipulating multiple processes at one time and keeping information in working memory (in math) • Test taking: Repeats the same errors on tests • Poor self-checking	• Procedure lists (breaking procedures down into numbered steps) • Metacognitive questions and prompts • Personalized checklists for common errors • "Give it the ONCE over" for math (Operations, Numbers, Calculation, Estimation) • "Top Three Hits" (personalized checklist)	• Teacher allows and encourages students to refer to their strategy notebooks and personalized checklists on tests • Teacher allocates additional time to check and correct work • Time reserved for "strategy-sharing" discussions and reflections about learning, self-monitoring, and learning styles

CASE 4

David, 17-Year-Old 12th Grader
*Executive Function Weaknesses That Affect
Organizing, Planning, Prioritizing*

BACKGROUND

David is an outgoing high school senior with no diagnosed learning or attention difficulties. He performed well in elementary and middle school; however, the increase in complexity and volume of his academic workload has exposed weaknesses in his executive function processes, especially organization and planning. During the past year, he has had particular difficulty staying focused in required classes that are not inherently interesting to him. His notes on lectures and readings have been disorganized, and he has also lacked a consistent method of studying for his exams. When studying, he has been staying up late the night before an exam, spending many hours rereading his textbook and looking over his notes. As a result, his grades over the past year have fluctuated from A's to D's. Due to his procrastination and difficulty with initiating tasks, he has also turned in many of his papers late this year. In an effort to improve David's time management and study skills, his school counselor has advised him to attend study skills sessions after school, in addition to weekly educational therapy.

RECOMMENDATIONS

Working with his educational therapist, David has begun to set measurable, attainable goals and to reward himself when he follows through. To avoid procrastination, he has learned how to break down large tasks into manageable steps and to prioritize. David now uses time estimation worksheets to increase his awareness of how much time he needs to complete his work. He has also learned several strategies for note taking and active studying which help him to synthesize information instead of just "glancing over" the reading material and his notes. For example, he has learned to "Read, Reflect, and Write"—that is, first to *read* a section of the text, then to *reflect* on what is important, and then to *write* it down. He uses Triple Note Tote (see Chapters 2 and 4) to organize information, making it readily available for studying before tests. In addition, while reading and studying, he now underlines and indents his notes so that he can differentiate between main ideas and details. These strategies, all compiled and recorded in a strategy notebook, have helped David to study more effectively and to improve his grades. Table III.4 summarizes the recommended strategies and accommodations for David.

TABLE III.4. David, 17-Year-Old 12th Grader

Executive function weaknesses	Educational difficulties	Recommended strategies	Accommodations
Organizing, prioritizing	• Inefficient study skills; often simply glances over materials • Poor note-taking strategies; messy notes • Difficulty attending to details when reading • Test taking: Poor grades on exams	• Strategies for note taking and active reading (e.g., Read, Reflect, Write; Triple Note Tote; margin notes and highlighting) • Strategies for making notes more visually organized: skipping lines, indenting, underlining, using bullets • Strategy notebook	• Teacher requires submission of study plan • Teacher provides feedback on note taking • Teacher requires use of strategy reflection sheets and allocates part of the grade for strategy use • Study skills support
Planning, prioritizing	• Difficulty with time management • Procrastinates—leaves tasks until last minute • Constant feeling of being overwhelmed with work	• Strategies for goal setting (long-term and short-term) and for breaking down tasks • Time estimation worksheets • Monthly and weekly calendars, "to-do" lists, planning sheets • Rewards himself for meeting goals	• Submission of goal-setting and time estimation worksheets required by teacher • Teacher provides opportunities for setting goals • Teacher allows time for discussions on goal setting and strategy use • Teacher allows time and provides calendar for long-term planning

APPENDIX

REPRODUCIBLES FOR THE CLASSROOM

Individual Goal Plain

My goal is

My target date is

To reach my goal, I will do these three things:

1.

2.

3.

I will know I've reached my goal when _____

_____

_____

Two things that will help me stick to my goal are:

1.

2.

If I run into problems, I can do these two things:

1.

2.

Individual Goal-Planning Worksheet

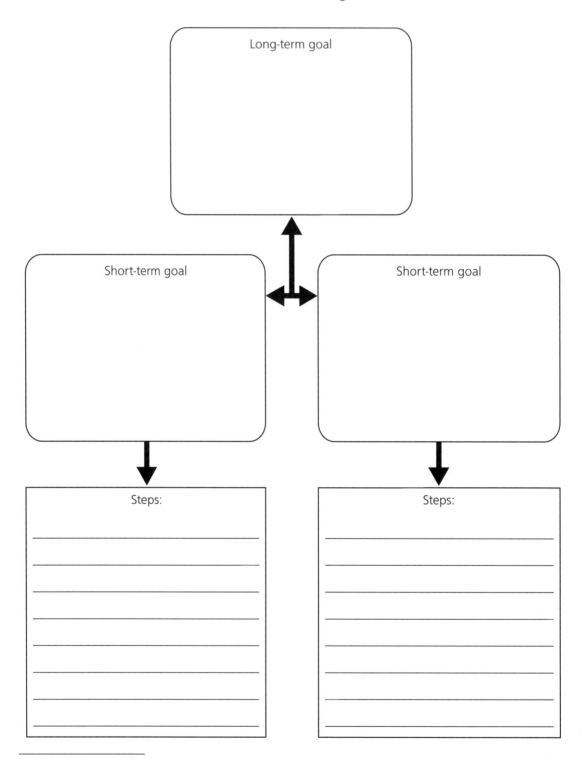

Time Estimation Worksheet

When do you lose track of time? Mark the appropriate place on the line. Keep in mind that a distraction is anything you are doing besides watching the clock.

<--->

| After 1 minute with distraction | After 5 minutes with distraction | After 10 minutes with distraction | After 15 minutes with distraction | After 20 minutes with distraction |

Now I know that after _____ minutes I need to use:

☐ An egg timer

☐ A microwave timer

☐ A helpful parent or sibling

☐ A visual time tracker or clock

Strategy Reflection Sheet

(Strategy Reflection)

Task:

Strategy:

Did your organizing strategy work well?

Why or why not?

Sorting and Categorizing in the Content Areas
How Can We Group Them?

Work with your team members to sort your group of items, pictures, or words into three to six categories. Write your answers in the boxes below. Then fill out your reflection.

Category Name:

Category Name:

Category Name:

Category Name:

Category Name:

Category Name:

Character Traits Sheet

Character	Important Trait	Evidence from Novel

From *Promoting Executive Function in the Classroom* by Lynn Meltzer. Copyright 2010 by The Guilford Press. Permission to photocopy this form is granted to purchasers of this book for personal use only (see copyright page for details).

Crazy Phrase Strategy Template for Remembering

Crazy phrase: A made-up silly sentence to help you remember sequential information.

When: Helpful when you need to remember names, places, events or operations in a specific order (e.g., planets in the solar system, countries on a map, steps in long division).

How:
1. List the information in order.
2. Write the first letter from each word.
3. Create a silly sentence whose words begin with these letters. Try to make up a sentence that creates a funny picture in your head.
4. Rehearse the sentence until you remember it easily.

List the information:	Write the first letters:	Create a crazy phrase:

Don't forgot to rehearse the sentence! Drawing a cartoon of your crazy phrase can be a powerful memory tool too.

Chapter Summary Organizer

Title: _____

Chapter: _____

Setting: _____

Characters: _____

   Main character's name: _____

   Three facts about the main character:

     1. _____

     2. _____

     3. _____

Have you learned anything new about the main character's problem? Write it down.

Summary (write down the most important thing that occurred in this chapter):

New vocabulary form this chapter:

KNOW Strategy Template for Doing Word Problems

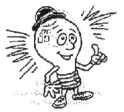

"I Know how to do
word problems!"

Name: _____

Date: _____

Key words or phrases

Numbers that I need

Operation(s)

Work it out!

Steinberg, J.
© ResearchILD 2005

RAPS Strategy Template for Breaking Down
Parts of a Word Problem

Name: _____

Date: _____

Read and Rephrase

Art

Plan and Predict

Solve

© ResearchILD 2005

How Do the Details Support the Main Idea?

Main Idea:	Main Idea:	Main Idea:
It shows that . . .	It shows that . . .	It shows that . . .
Detail:	Detail:	Detail:

Guide for Making Revisions to a Five-Paragraph Essay

Question	Yes or No?	Action Steps
Is there a thesis statement?		Add one or two sentences that summarize your viewpoint or main idea.
Is the essay organized into paragraphs?		Divide essay into introduction, three body paragraphs, and conclusion.
Is there an introduction?		Write a paragraph that introduces your topic and includes a thesis.
Does each body paragraph have a topic sentence?		Add a sentence that introduces the topic of each paragraph.
Does the essay contain sufficient supporting details?		Add more quotes, facts, or specific examples to body paragraphs.
Is there a conclusion?		Add a paragraph that summarizes your opinion or main idea.
Does the essay flow well and read smoothly?		Use transition words to link sentences and paragraphs.
Does the essay contain colorful and interesting vocabulary?		Replace common words with ones that are more vivid and unusual.

APPENDIX 13

Personalized Checking Cards for Tests

Checking Card for Multiple-Choice Tests

Did I . . .

- ☐ Write my name and the date on the test?
- ☐ Underline key words in each question (e.g., *except for*)?
- ☐ Circle only one answer for each question?
- ☐ Answer all the questions on the test?

For questions I am unsure of, did I . . .

- ☐ Read the question carefully and pay attention to key words?
- ☐ Eliminate obviously incorrect answers?
- ☐ Choose the answer that seems the most logical from the remaining possibilities?

Checking Card for Essay Tests

Did I . . .

- ☐ Write my name and the date on the test?
- ☐ Underline key words in the question (e.g., *compare, contrast*)?
- ☐ Use a prewriting strategy (e.g., outline, web/map)?
- ☐ Include an introduction, body paragraphs, and conclusion?
- ☐ Add enough details and specific examples?
- ☐ Use a proofreading strategy (e.g., acronym or checklist)?

References

Adelman, H. S., & Taylor, L. (1993). *Learning problems and learning disabilities: Moving forward*. Pacific Grove, CA: Brooks/Cole.

Alexander, P. A. (1998). The nature of disciplinary and domain learning: The knowledge, interest, and strategic dimensions of learning from subject matter text. In C. R. Hynd (Ed.), *Learning from text across conceptual domains* (pp. 263–286). Mahwah, NJ: Erlbaum.

Alexander, P. A. (2004). A model of domain learning: Reinterpreting expertise as a multidimensional, multistage process. In D. Yun Dai & R. J. Sternberg (Eds.), *Motivation, emotion, and cognition: Integrative perspectives on intellectual functioning and development* (pp. 273–299). Mahwah, NJ: Erlbaum.

Alexander, P. A., & Murphy, P. K. (1998). Profiling the differences in students' knowledge, interest, and strategic processing. *Journal of Educational Psychology, 90*, 435–477.

Anderson, V., Rani Jacobs, J., & Anderson, P. (Eds.) (2008). *Executive functions and the frontal lobes: A lifespan perspective*. New York: Taylor and Francis.

Andrews, G., & Halford, G. S. (2002). A cognitive complexity metric applied to cognitive development. *Cognitive Psychology, 45*, 153–219.

Baddeley, A. (2006). Working memory: An overview. In S. Pickering (Ed.), *Working memory and education* (pp. 3–26). Boston: Academic Press.

Baerveldt, A., Madison, A., & Martinussen, R. (2008, June). *Cognitive and academic correlates of report writing in elementary-age children*. Paper presented at the 32nd Annual Conference of the International Academy for Research in Learning Disabilities, Toronto.

Bandura, A. (1986). *Social foundations of thought and action: A social cognitive theory*. Englewood Cliffs, NJ: Prentice-Hall.

Barkley, R. A., Copeland, A. P., & Sivage, C. (1980). A self-control classroom for hyperactive children. *Journal of Autism and Developmental Disorders, 10*, 75–89.

Barlow, D. H. (2000). Unraveling the mysteries of anxiety and its disorders from the perspective of emotion theory. *American Psychologist, 55*(11), 1245–1263.

Begley, S. (2007). *Train your mind, change your brain: How a new science reveals our extraordinary potential to transform ourselves.* New York: Ballantine Books.

Bell, N. (1986). *Visualizing and verbalizing for language comprehension.* San Luis Obispo, CA: Gander Educational.

Bereiter, C., & Scardamalia, M. (1993). *Surpassing ourselves: An inquiry into the nature and implications of expertise.* Chicago: Open Court.

Berninger, V. W., Abbott, R., Thomson, J., & Raskind, W. (2001). Language phenotype for reading and writing disability: A family approach. *Scientific Studies in Reading, 5,* 59–105.

Berninger, V. W., & Nagy, W. E. (2008). Flexibility in word reading: Multiple levels of representations, complex mappings, partial similarities, and cross-modality connections. In K. B. Cartwright (Ed.), *Literacy processes: Cognitive flexibility in learning and teaching* (pp. 114–142). New York: Guilford Press.

Bernstein, J., & Waber, D. (2007). Executive capacities from a developmental perspective. In L. Meltzer (Ed.) *Executive function in education: From theory to practice.* (pp. 39–54). New York: Guilford Press.

Black, B. (1995). *The Reach Out to Schools social competency program: Assessment summary.* Unpublished manuscript, The Stone Center, Wellesley College.

Block, C. C., & Pressley, M. (Eds.). (2002). *Comprehension instruction: Research-based best practices.* New York: Guilford Press.

Booth, S. R., & Fairbank, D. W. (1983). Videotaped feedback as a behavior management technique. *Behavioral Disorders, 9,* 55–59.

Bos, C. S., & Anderson, P. L. (1990). Effects of interactive vocabulary instruction on vocabulary learning and reading comprehension of junior-high learning disabled students. *Learning Disability Quarterly, 13,* 31–42.

Bos, C. S., & Vaughn, S. (2002). *Strategies for teaching students with learning and behavior problems.* Boston: Allyn & Bacon.

Bransford, J., Brown, A., & Cocking, R. (Eds.). (2000). *How people learn: Brain, mind, experience, and school.* Washington, DC: National Academy Press.

Bransford, J. D., & Johnson, M. K. (1973). Consideration of some problems in comprehension. In W. G. Chase (Ed.), *Visual information processing* (pp. 383–   438). New York: Academic Press.

Bremer, C. D., Vaughn, S., Clapper, A. T., & Kim, A. (2002). Collaborative strategic reading (CSR): Improving secondary students' reading comprehension skills. *Research to Practice Brief, 1*(2), 1–9.

Bridges, L. J., Margie, N. G., & Zaff, F. J. (2001, December). *Background for community-level work in emotional well-being in adolescence: Reviewing the literature on contributing factors* (Child Trends Research Brief). Washington, DC: John S. and James L. Knight Foundation.

Britton, B., & Tesser, A. (1991). Effects of time-management practices on college grads. *Journal of Educational Psychology, 83*(3), 405–410.

Bronfenbrenner, U. (1979). Contexts of child rearing: Problems and prospects. *American Psychologist, 34*(10), 844–850.

Brooks, R. (1991). *The self-esteem teacher: Seeds of self-esteem.* New York: Treehaus.

Brown, A. L. (1997). Transforming schools into communities of thinking and learning about serious matters. *American Psychologist, 52*(4), 399–413.

Brown, A. L., Bransford, J. D., Ferrara, R. A., & Campione, J. (1983). Learning, remembering and understanding. In P. H. Mussen (Series Ed.) & E. M. Hetherington (Vol. Ed.), *Handbook of child psychology: Vol. 4. Socialization, personality, and social development* (4th ed., pp. 77–166). New York: Wiley.

Brown, A. L., & Campione, J. C. (1986). Psychological theory and the study of learning disabilities. *American Psychologist, 41*(10), 1059–1068.

Brown, G. D. A., & Deavers, R. P. (1999). Units of analysis in nonword reading: Evidence from children and adults. *Journal of Experimental Child Psychology, 73*, 203–242.

Bruning, R., & Horn, R. (2000). Developing motivation to write. *Educational Psychologist, 35*(1), 25–38.

Brunstein, J. C., Schultheiss, O. C., & Grässmann, R. (1998). Personal goals and emotional well-being: The moderating role of motive dispositions. *Journal of Personality and Social Psychology, 75*(2), 494–508.

Buehler, R., Griffin, D., & MacDonald, H. (1997). The role of motivated reasoning in optimistic time predictions. *Personality and Social Psychology Bulletin, 23*, 238–247.

Bull, R., & Scerif, G. (2001). Executive functioning as a predictor of children's mathematics ability: Inhibition, switching, and working memory. *Developmental Neuropsychology, 19*, 273–293.

Caine, G., & Caine, R. N. (2006). Meaningful learning and the executive functions of the brain. *New Directions for Adult and Continuing Education, 110*, 53–61.

Carlson, C. L., Booth, J. E., Shin, M., & Canu, W. H. (2002). Parent, teacher, and self-rated motivational styles in ADHD subtypes. *Journal of Learning Disabilities, 35*(2), 104–113.

Carney, R. N., Levin, M. E., & Levin, J. R. (1993). Mnemonic strategies: Instructional techniques worth remembering. *Teaching Exceptional Children, 25*(4), 24–30.

Cartwright, K. B. (2002). Cognitive development and reading: The relation of multiple classification skill to reading comprehension in elementary school children. *Journal of Educational Psychology, 94*, 56–63.

Cartwright, K. B. (Ed.). (2008a). *Literacy processes: Cognitive flexibility in learning and teaching.* New York: Guilford Press.

Cartwright, K. B. (2008b). Introduction to literacy processes: Cognitive flexibility in learning and teaching. In K. B. Cartwright (Ed.), *Literacy processes: Cognitive flexibility in learning and teaching* (pp. 3–18). New York: Guilford Press.

Cartwright, K. B. (2008c). Concluding reflections: What can we learn from considering implications of representational development and flexibility for literacy teaching and learning? In K. B. Cartwright (Ed.), *Literacy processes: Cognitive flexibility in learning and teaching* (pp. 359–371). New York: Guilford Press.

Cole, P., Martin, S., & Dennis, T. (2004). Emotional regulation as a scientific construct: Methodological challenges and directions for child development research. *Child Development, 75*(2), 317–333.

Combs, M. (1996). *Developing competent readers and writers in the primary grades.* Englewood Cliffs, NJ: Prentice-Hall.

Cushman, K. (1998). *The ballad of Lucy Whipple.* New York: Harper Trophy.

Daneman, M., & Carpenter, P. (1980). Individual differences in working memory and reading. *Journal of Verbal Learning and Verbal Behavior, 19*(4), 450–466.

Deák, G. O. (2008). Foreword. In K. B. Cartwright (Ed.), *Literacy processes: Cognitive flexibility in learning and teaching.* New York: Guilford Press.

Deci, E. L., & Ryan, R. M. (1985). *Intrinsic motivation and self-determination in human behavior.* New York: Plenum Press.

Deci, E. L., & Ryan, R. M. (2000). The 'what' and 'why' of goal pursuits: Human needs and the self-determination of behavior. *Psychological Inquiry, 11*(4), 227–268.

de Fockert, J. W., Rees, G., Frith, C. D., & Lavie, N. (2001). The role of working memory in visual selective attention. *Science, 291*(5509), 1803–1806.

De La Paz, S. (2007). Best practices in teaching writing to students with special needs. In S. Graham, C. A. McArthur, & J. Fitzgerald (Eds.), *Best practices in writing instruction* (pp. 308–328). New York: Guilford Press.

De La Paz, S., & Graham, S. (1997). Effects of dictation and advanced planning instruction on the composing of students with writing and learning problems. *Journal of Educational Psychology, 89,* 203–222.

Denckla, M. B. (2005). Executive function. In D. Gozal & D. Molfese (Eds.), *Attention deficit hyperactivity disorder: From genes to patients* (pp. 165–183). Totowa, NJ: Humana Press.

Denckla, M. (2007). Executive function: Binding together the definitions of attention deficit/hyperactivity disorder and learning disabilities. In L. Meltzer (Ed.) *Executive function on Education: From theory to practice* (pp. 5–18). New York: Guilford Press.

Denckla, M. B. (2007). Executive function: Binding together the definitions of attention deficit/hyperactivity disorder and learning disabilities. In L. Meltzer (Ed.), *Executive function in education: From theory to practice* (pp. 5–19). New York: Guilford Press.

Deshler, D. D., Ellis, E. S., & Lenz, B. K. (Eds.). (1996). *Teaching adolescents with learning disabilities: Strategies and methods* (2nd ed.). Denver, CO: Love.

Deshler, D. D., & Schumaker, J. B. (1988). An instructional model for teaching students how to learn. In J. L. Graden, J. E. Zins, & M. J. Curtis (Eds.), *Alternative education delivery systems: Enhancing instructional options for all students* (pp. 391–411). Washington, DC: National Association of School Psychologists.

Deshler, D. D., Schumaker, J. B., & Lenz, B. K. (1984). Academic and cognitive interventions for LD adolescents. *Journal of Learning Disabilities, 17*(33), 170–179.

Deshler, D. D., Schumaker, J. B., Lenz, B. K., Bulgren, J., Hock, M., Knight, J., et al. (2001). Ensuring content-area learning by secondary students with learning disabilities. *Learning Disabilities Research and Practice, 16*(2), 96–108.

Diamond, A. (2006). The early development of executive functions. In E. Bialystok & F. Craik (Eds.), *Lifespan cognition: Mechanisms of change* (pp. 70–95). New York: Oxford University Press.

Doll, B., Zucker, S., & Brehm, K. (2004). *Resilient classrooms: Creating healthy environments for learning.* New York: Guilford Press.

Dunlap, L. K., & Dunlap, G. (1989). A self-monitoring package for teaching subtraction with regrouping to students with learning disabilities. *Journal of Applied Behavior Analysis, 22*(3), 309–314.

Dweck, C. S. (2006). *Mindset: The new psychology of success.* New York: Random House.

Dweck, C. C., & Molden, D. (2005). Self-theories: Their impact on competence motivation and acquisition. In A. J. Eliot & C. S. Dweck (Eds.) *Handbook of competence and motivation* (pp. 122–140). New York: Guilford Press.

Eccles, J. S. (1987). Gender roles and women's achievement-related decisions. *Psychology of Women Quarterly, 11,* 135–173.

Eggen, P. D., & Kauchak, D. (1992). *Educational psychology: Classroom connections.* New York: Macmillan.

Ehri, L. C. (1991). Learning to read and spell words. In L. Rieben & C. A. Perfetti (Eds.), *Learning to read: Basic research and its implications* (pp. 57–74). Hillsdale, NJ: Erlbaum.

Elliot, A. J., & Dweck, C. S. (2005). Competence and motivation: Competence as the core of achievement motivation. In A. J. Elliot & C. S. Dweck (Eds.), *Handbook of competence and motivation* (pp. 3–15). New York: Guilford Press.

Ellis, E. S. (1997). Watering up the curriculum for adolescents with learning disabilities: Goals of the knowledge dimension. *Remedial and Special Education, 18,* 326–346.

Enfield, M. L., & Greene, V. (1989). *Project Read original evaluation/research summary: 1969–1989.* Retrieved May 20, 2009, from *www.projectread.com*

Englert, C., Raphael, T., & Anderson, L. (1992). Socially-mediated instruction: Improving students' knowledge and talk about writing. *Elementary School Journal, 92,* 411–447.

Feather, N. T. (1988). Values, valence, and course enrollment: Testing the role of personal values within an expectancy–value framework. *Journal of Educational Psychology, 80,* 380–391.

Fishbein, M., & Ajzen, I. (1975). *Belief, attitude, intention, and behavior: An introduction to theory and research.* Reading, MA: Addison-Wesley.

Flavell, J. H. (1979). Metacognition and cognitive monitoring: A new area of cognitive-developmental inquiry. *American Psychologist, 34,* 906–911.

Flower, L., Stein, V., Ackerman, J., Kantz, M. J., McCormick, K., & Peck, W. C. (1990). *Reading-to-write: Exploring a cognitive and social process.* New York: Oxford University Press.

Flower, L., Wallace, D. L., Norris, L., & Burnett, R. A. (1994). *Making thinking visible: Writing, collaborative planning, and classroom inquiry.* Urbana, IL: National Council of Teachers of English.

Fry, E. B. (1978). *Skimming and scanning.* Providence, RI: Jamestown.

Fuchs, D., & Fuchs, L. S. (1991). Framing the REI debate: Conservationists vs. abolitionists. In J. W. Lloyd, N. N. Singh, & A. C. Repp (Eds.), *The regular education initiative: Alternative perspectives on concepts, issues, and models* (pp. 241–255). DeKalb, IL: Sycamore.

Fuchs, D., Fuchs, L. S., & Burish, P. (2000). Peer-assisted learning strategies: An evidence based practice to promote reading achievement. *Learning Disabilities Research and Practice, 15*(2), 85–91.

Fuchs, L. S., Fuchs, D., & Deno, S. L. (1985). Importance of goal ambitiousness and goal mastery to student achievement. *Exceptional Children, 52,* 63–71.

Gardner, H. (1983). *Frames of mind: The theory of multiple intelligences.* New York: Basic Books.

Gaskins, I. W. (2008). Developing cognitive flexibility in word reading among beginning and struggling readers. In K. B. Cartwright (Ed.), *Literacy processes: Cognitive flexibility in learning and teaching* (pp. 90–114). New York: Guilford Press.

Gaskins, I. W., & Pressley, M. (2007). Teaching metacognitive strategies that address executive function processes within a schoolwide curriculum. In L. Meltzer (Ed.), *Executive function in education: From theory to practice* (pp. 261–286). New York: Guilford Press.

Gaskins, I. W., Satlow, E., & Pressley, M. (2007). Executive control of reading comprehension in the elementary school. In L. Meltzer (Ed.), *Executive function in education: From theory to practice* (pp. 194–216). New York: Guilford Press.

Gathercole, S., Lamont, E., & Alloway, T. P. (2006). Working memory in the classroom. In S. Pickering (Ed.), *Working memory and education* (pp. 220–238). Boston: Academic Press.

Gendlin, E. T. (1981). *Focusing.* New York: Bantam Books.

Gettinger, M., & Seibert, J. K. (2002). Effective study skills promote positive outcomes across subject areas. *Psychology Review, 13*(3), 350–365.

Gibson, E. (2006). *How to remember everything: Memory shortcuts to help you study smarter, grades 6–8.* New York: Random House.

Gioia, G. A., Isquith, P. K., Guy, S. C., & Kenworthy, L. (2000). *Behavior Rating Inventory of Executive Function.* Odessa, FL: Psychological Assessment Resources.

Gioia, G. A., Isquith, P. K., Kenworthy, L., & Barton, R. (2002). Profiles of everyday executive function in acquired and developmental disorders. *Child Neuropsychology, 8*(2), 121–137.

Goldstein, S., & Brooks, B. (Eds.). (2005). *Handbook of resilience in children.* Cambridge, MA: Birkhauser.

Goleman, D. (1995). *Emotional intelligence.* New York: Bantam Books.

Goswami, U., Ziegler, J. C., Dalton, L., & Schneider, W. (2001). Pseudohomophone effects and phonological recoding procedures in reading development in English and German. *Journal of Memory and Language, 45,* 648–664.

Goswami, U., Ziegler, J. C., Dalton, L., & Schneider, W. (2003). Nonword reading across orthographies: How flexible is the choice of reading units? *Applied Psycholinguistics, 24,* 235–247.

Graham, S. (1990). The role of production factors in learning disabled students' compositions. *Journal of Educational Psychology, 82,* 781–791.

Graham, S. (2006). Writing. In P. A. Alexander & P. H. Winnie (Eds.), *Handbook of educational psychology* (pp. 457–478). Mahwah, NJ: Erlbaum.

Graham, S., & Harris, K. R. (1989). Improving learning disabled students' skills at composing essays: Self-instructional strategy training. *Exceptional Children, 56,* 201–214.

Graham, S., & Harris, K. R. (2003). Students with learning disabilities and the process of writing: A meta-analysis of SRSD studies. In H. L. Swanson, K. R. Harris, & S. Graham (Eds.), *Handbook of learning disabilities* (pp. 383–402). New York: Guilford Press.

Graham, S., & Harris, K. R. (2005). *Writing better: Effective strategies for teaching students with learning difficulties.* Baltimore: Brookes.

Graham, S., Harris, K. R., & Olinghouse, N. (2007a). Addressing executive function problems in writing: An example from the self-regulated strategy development model. In L. Meltzer (Ed.), *Executive function in education: From theory to practice* (pp. 216–236). New York: Guilford Press.

Graham, S., MacArthur, C. A., & Fitzgerald, J. (Eds.). (2007b). *Best practices in writing instruction.* New York: Guilford Press.

Gray, L. (2007). *Islands of confidence: The impact of the SMARTS mentoring program on the self-concepts and success attributes of a sample of young adults with learning and attention difficulties.* Unpublished manuscript, Middlebury College.

Gray, L., Meltzer, C., & Upton, M. (2008, March). *The SMARTS peer mentoring program: Fostering self-understanding and resilience across the grades.* Paper presented at the 23rd Annual Learning Differences Conference, Harvard Graduate School of Education, Cambridge, MA.

Greenberg, M. T., Kusche, C. A., Cook E. T., & Quamma, J. P. (1995). Promoting emotional competence in school-aged children: The effects of the PATHS curriculum. *Development and Psychopathology, 7,* 117–136.

Gross, J. J. (1998). The emerging field of emotion regulation: An integrative review. *Review of General Psychology, 2,* 271–299.

Gross, J. J. (Ed.). (2007). *Handbook of emotion regulation.* New York: Guilford Press.

Gross, J. J., & Thompson, R. A. (2007). Emotion regulation: Conceptual foundations. In J. J. Gross (Ed.), *Handbook of emotion regulation* (pp. 3–26). New York: Guilford Press.

Hallowell, E. M., & Ratey, J. J. (1994). *Driven to distraction: Recognizing and coping with attention deficit hyperactivity disorder from childhood through adulthood.* New York: Random House.

Harris, K. R., & Graham, S. (1992). *Helping young writers master the craft: Strategy instruction and self-regulation in the writing process.* Cambridge, MA: Brookline Books.

Harris, K. R., & Graham, S. (1996). *Making the writing process work: Strategies for composition and self-regulation.* Cambridge, MA: Brookline Books.

Harris, K. R., Graham, S., & Mason, L. H. (2003). Self-regulated strategy development in the classroom: Part of a balanced approach to writing instruction for students with disabilities. *Focus on Exceptional Children, 35*(7), 1–16.

Harris, K. R., Graham, S., Mason, L. H., & Friedlander, B. (2008). *Powerful writing strategies for all students.* Baltimore: Brookes.

Harris, K. R., & Pressley, M. (1991). The nature of cognitive strategy instruction: Interactive strategy instruction. *Exceptional Children, 57,* 392–403.

Hattie, J., Biggs, J., & Purdie, N. (1996). Effects of learning skills interventions on student learning: A meta-analysis. *Review of Educational Research, 66*(2), 99–136.

Hawkins, J. D., & Catalano R. F. (1992). *Communities that care: Action for drug abuse prevention.* San Francisco: Jossey-Bass.

Helliwell, J. F. (2003). How's life?: Combing individual and national variations to explain subjective well being. *Economic Modeling, 20,* 331–360.

Hennessey, B. A. (2007). Promoting social competence in school-aged children: The effects of the open circle program. *Journal of School Psychology, 45,* 349–360.

Hidi, S., Renninger, K. A., & Krapp, A. (2004). Interest, a motivational variable that combines affective and cognitive functioning. In D. Yun Dai & R. J. Sternberg (Eds.), *Motivation, emotion, and cognition: Integrative perspectives on intellectual functioning and development* (pp. 89–115). Mahwah, NJ: Erlbaum.

Higbee, K. L. (1988). *Your memory: How it works and how to improve it.* London: Piatkus.

Goldman-Rakic, P. (1992). Working memory and the mind. *Scientific American, 267*(3), 110–117.

Holmes Bernstein, J., & Waber, D. (2007). Executive capabilities from a developmental perspective. In L. Meltzer (Ed.), *Executive function on Education: From theory to practice* (pp. 39–54). New York: Guilford Press.

Homer, B. D., & Hayward, E. O. (2008). Cognitive and representational development in children. In K. B. Cartwright (Ed.), *Literacy processes: Cognitive flexibility in learning and teaching* (pp. 19–42). New York: Guilford Press.

Hongwanishkul, D., Happaney, K. R., Lee, W. S., & Zelazo, D. (2005). Assessment of hot and cool executive function in young children: Age-related changes and individual differences. *Developmental Neuropsychology, 28*(2), 617–644.

Hughes, C. (1996). Memory and test-taking strategies. In D. D. Deshler, E. S. Ellis, & B. K. Lenz (Eds.), *Teaching adolescents with learning disabilities: Strategies and methods* (2nd ed., pp. 209–266). Denver, CO: Love.

Huttenlocher, P. R., & Dabholkar, A. S. (1997). Developmental anatomy of prefrontal cortex. In N. A. Krasnegor, G. R. Lyon, & P. S. Goldman-Rakic (Eds.), *Development of the prefrontal cortex: Evolution, neurobiology and behavior* (pp. 69–83). Baltimore: Brookes.

Jennings, T., & Haynes, C. (2002). *From talking to writing: Strategies for scaffolding expository expression*. Prides Crossing, MA: Landmark School.

John, O., & Gross, J. J. (2007). Individual differences in emotional regulation. In J. J. Gross (Ed.), *Handbook of emotional regulation* (pp. 351–372). New York: Guilford Press.

Johnson, L., Graham, S., & Harris, K. (1997). The effects of goal setting and self-instruction on learning a reading comprehension strategy: A study of students with learning disabilities. *Journal of Learning Disabilities, 30,* 80–91.

Joseph, N. L. (2003). *Metacognitive awareness: Investigating theory and practice.* Retrieved December 3, 2008, from *www.thefreelibrary.com/Metacognitive+awareness:+investigating+theory+and+practice-a0114168082*

Josephs, R., & Hahn, E. (1995). Bias and accuracy in estimates of task duration. *Organizational Behavior and Human Decision Processes, 61,* 202–213.

Kagan, J. (1989). *Unstable ideas: Temperament, cognition, and self.* Cambridge, MA: Harvard University Press.

Kame'enui, E. (2007). A new paradigm: Responsiveness to intervention. *Teaching Exceptional Children, 39*(5), 6–8.

Kasser, T., & Ryan, R. M. (1996). Further examining the American dream: Differential correlates of intrinsic and extrinsic goals. *Personality and Social Psychology Bulletin, 22,* 280–287.

Kendall, P. C., & Zupan, B. A. (1981). Individual versus group application of cognitive-behavioral self-control procedures with children. *Behavioral Therapy, 12,* 344–359.

Klingner, J. K., & Vaughn, S. (1996). Reciprocal teaching of reading comprehension strategies for students with learning disabilities who use English as a second language. *Elementary School Journal, 96*(3), 275–293.

Klingner, J. K., Vaughn, S., & Boardman, A. (2007). *Teaching reading comprehension to students with learning difficulties.* New York: Guilford Press.

Kops, C., & Belmont, I. (1985). Planning and organizing skills of poor school achievers. *Journal of Learning Disabilities, 18*(1), 8–14.

Kotelf, B. J., & Seigle, P. (2006). Inside Open Circle. In M. J. Elias & H. Arnold (Eds.), *The educator's guide to emotional intelligence and academic achievement social-emotional learning in the classroom* (pp. 140–149). Thousand Oaks, CA: Corwin Press.

Kwane-Ross, T. (2003, Winter). In just a minute: Teaching students the skills of waiting. *Responsive Classroom Newsletter, 15*(1), 1–4.

Levine, P., & Kline, M. (2006). *Trauma through a child's eyes.* Berkeley, CA: North Atlantic Books.

Licht, B. G. (1983). Cognitive-motivational factors that contribute to the achievement of learning-disabled children. *Journal of Learning Disabilities, 16,* 483–490.

Licht, B. G. (1993). Achievement-related believes in children with learning disabilities: Impact on motivation and strategic learning. In L. Meltzer (Ed.), *Strategy assessment and instruction for students with learning disabilities: From theory to practice* (pp. 195–220). Austin, TX: PRO-ED.

Linskie, R. (1977). *The learning process: Theory and practice.* New York: Van Nostrand.

Locke, E. A. (1968). Towards a theory of task motivation and incentives. *Organizational Behavior and Human Performance, 3,* 157–189.

Locke, E. A., Shaw, K. N., Saari, L. M., & Latham, G. P. (1981). Goal setting and task performance: 1969–1980. *Psychological Bulletin, 90*(1), 125–152.

Lovett, M. W., Lacerenza, L., & Borden, S. (2000). Putting struggling readers on the PHAST track: A program to integrate phonological and strategy-based remedial reading instruction and maximize outcomes. *Journal of Learning Disabilities, 33*, 458–476.

MacArthur, C., Graham, S., & Fitzgerald, J. (Eds.). (2006). *Handbook of writing research.* New York: Guilford Press.

Maccini, P., & Hughes, C. A. (1997). Mathematics interventions for adolescents with learning disabilities. *Learning Disabilities Research and Practice, 12*(3), 168–176.

Macklem, G. L. (2008). *Practitioner's guide to emotion regulation in school-aged children.* New York: Springer Science + Business Media.

Marlowe, W. (2000). An intervention for children with disorders of executive functions. *Developmental Neuropsychology, 18*(3), 445–454.

Marmorstein, N. R. (2007). Relationships between anxiety and externalizing disorders in youth: The influence of age and gender. *Journal of Anxiety Disorders, 21*, 420–432.

Marzano, R. J. (2003). *What works in schools: Translating research into action.* Alexandria, VA: Association for Supervision and Curriculum Development.

Massey, D. (2008). Teaching flexibility?: Possibilities and challenges. In K. B. Cartwright (Ed.), *Literacy processes: Cognitive flexibility in learning and teaching* (pp. 300–320). New York: Guilford Press.

Mastropieri, M. A., & Scruggs, T. E. (1991). *Teaching students ways to remember: Strategies for learning mnemonically.* Cambridge, MA: Brookline Books.

Mastropieri, M. A., & Scruggs, T. E. (1995). Teaching science to students with disabilities in general education settings. *Teaching Exceptional Children, 27*, 10–13.

Mastropieri, M. A., & Scruggs, T. E. (1998). Enhancing school success with mnemonic strategies. *Intervention in School and Clinic, 33*, 201–208.

Mastropieri, M. A., & Scruggs, T. E. (2000). *The inclusive classroom: Strategies for effective instruction.* Upper Saddle River, NJ: Merrill.

Mastropieri, M. A., Scruggs, T., Mohler, L., Beranek, M., Spencer, V., Boon, R. T., et al. (2001). Can middle school students with serious reading difficulties help each other and learn anything? *Learning Disabilities Research and Practice, 16*(1), 18–27.

Mastropieri, M. A., Sweda, J., & Scruggs, T. E. (2000). Putting mnemonic strategies to work in an inclusive classroom. *Learning Disabilities Research and Practice, 15*(2), 69–74.

Matlin, M. W. (2002). *Cognition* (5th ed.). Fort Worth, TX: Harcourt College.

McNamara, D. S., & Scott, J. L. (2001). Working memory capacity and strategy use. *Memory & Cognition, 29*, 10–17.

Meltzer, L. (1993). Strategy use in children with learning disabilities: The challenge of assessment. In L. Meltzer (Ed.), *Strategy assessment and instruction for students with learning disabilities: From theory to practice* (pp. 93–136). Austin, TX: PRO-ED.

Meltzer, L. (1996). Strategic learning in students with learning disabilities: The role of self awareness and self-perception. In T. E. Scruggs & M. Mastropieri (Eds.), *Advances in learning and behavioral disabilities: Vol. 10b. Intervention research* (pp. 181–199). Greenwich, CT: JAI Press.

Meltzer, L. (2004). Resilience and learning disabilities: Research on internal and external protective dynamics. *Learning Disabilities Research and Practice, 19*(1), 1–2.

Meltzer, L. (Ed.). (2007). *Executive function in education: From theory to practice.* New York: Guilford Press.

Meltzer, L. (2008a, June). *Executive function strategies, effort, and self-efficacy: The keys to academic success*. Cruickshank Memorial Lecture presented at the 32nd Annual Conference of the International Academy for Research in Learning Disabilities, Toronto.

Meltzer, L. (2008b). *Executive function: Fostering strategic mindsets in the classroom*. Invited presentation at the 2008 Annual Convention of the Council for Exceptional Children, Boston.

Meltzer, L., Katzir, T., Miller, L., Reddy, R., & Roditi, B. (2004a). Academic self-perceptions, effort, and strategy use in students with learning disabilities: Changes over time. *Learning Disabilities Research and Practice, 19*(2), 99–108.

Meltzer, L., Katzir-Cohen, T., Miller, L., & Roditi, B. (2001). The impact of effort and strategy use on academic performance: Student and teacher perceptions. *Learning Disabilities Quarterly, 24*(2), 85–98.

Meltzer, L., & Krishnan, K. (2007). Executive function difficulties and learning disabilities: Understandings and misunderstandings. In L. Meltzer (Ed.), *Executive function in education: From theory to practice* (pp. 77–105). New York: Guilford Press.

Meltzer, L., & Montague, M. (2001). Strategic learning in students with learning disabilities: What have we learned? In B. Keogh & D. Hallahan (Eds.), *Intervention research and learning disabilities* (pp. 111–130). Hillsdale, NJ: Erlbaum.

Meltzer, L., Noeder, M., Basho, S., Stacey, W., Button, K., & Sales Pollica, L. (Chairs). (2007a, July). *Executive function strategies, effort, and academic self-perceptions: Impact on academic performance*. Symposium conducted at the 31st Annual Conference of the International Academy for Research in Learning Disabilities, Bled, Slovenia.

Meltzer, L., Sales Pollica, L., & Barzillai, M. (2007b). Executive function in the classroom: Embedding strategy instruction into daily teaching practices. In L. Meltzer (Ed.), *Executive function in education: From theory to practice* (pp. 165–193). New York: Guilford Press.

Meltzer, L., Reddy, R., Noeder, M., Basho, S., Stacey, W., & Button, K. (2010). *Promoting self-concept, effort, & executive function through peer tutoring*. Paper presented at the 34th Annual International Academy for Research in Learning Disabilities Conference, Miami, Florida.

Meltzer, L., Reddy, R., Sales Pollica, L., & Roditi, B. (2004b). Academic success in students with learning disabilities: The roles of self-understanding, strategy use, and effort. *Thalamus, 22*(1), 16–32.

Meltzer, L., Reddy, R., Sales Pollica, L., Roditi, B., Sayer, J., & Theokas, C. (2004c). Positive and negative self-perceptions: Is there a cyclical relationship between teachers' and students' perceptions of effort, strategy use, and academic performance? *Learning Disabilities Research and Practice, 19*(1), 33–44.

Meltzer, L., Roditi, B., Steinberg, J., Biddle, K., Taber, S., Caron, K., et al. (2006). *Strategies for success: Classroom teaching techniques for students with learning problems* (2nd ed.). Austin, TX: PRO-ED.

Meltzer, L., Sayer, J., Sales, L., Theokas, C., & Roditi, B. (2002, June). *Academic self perceptions in students with LD: Relationship with effort and strategy use*. Paper presented at the 26th Annual Conference of the International Academy for Research in Learning Disabilities, Washington, DC.

Meltzer, L., Solomon, B., Fenton, T., & Levine, M. D. (1989). A developmental study of problem-solving strategies in children with and without learning difficulties. *Journal of Applied Developmental Psychology, 10*, 171–193.

Miller, L., Meltzer, L., Katzir-Cohen, T., & Houser, R. F., Jr. (2001). Academic heterogeneity in students with learning disabilities. *Thalamus, 19*, 20–33.

Misra, R., & McKean, M. (2000). College students' academic stress and its relation to their anxiety, time management, and leisure satisfaction. *American Journal of Health Studies, 16*, 41–51.

Missiuna, C., Pollock, N., & Law, M. (2004). *The Perceived Efficacy and Goal Setting System.* San Antonio, TX: Psychological Corporation.

Missiuna, C., Pollock, N., Law, M., Walter, S., & Cavey, N. (2007). Examination of the Perceived Efficacy and Goal Setting System (PEGS) with children with disabilities, their parents, and teachers. *American Journal of Occupational Therapy, 60*(2), 204–214.

Montague, M. (2003). *Solve it: A mathematical problem-solving instructional program.* Reston, VA: Exceptional Innovations.

Montague, M., & Jitendra, A. K. (2006). *Teaching mathematics to middle school students with learning difficulties.* New York: Guilford Press.

Montague, M., Warger, C., & Morgan, H. (2000). Solve It!: Strategy instruction to improve mathematical problem solving. *Learning Disabilities Research and Practice, 15*, 110–116.

Moreau, M. E. R., & Fidrych-Puzzo, H. (2002). *How to use the Story Grammar Marker.* Springfield, MA: MindWing Concepts.

National Council of Teachers of Mathematics. (2000). *Principles and standards of math.* Reston: VA.

Nelson, R., Smith, D., & Dodd, J. (1992). The effects of teaching a summary skills strategy to students identified as learning disabled on their comprehension of science text. *Education and Treatment of Children, 15*, 228–243.

Noeder, M. (2007). *The Drive to Thrive program: Fostering effective strategy use, metacognitive awareness, effort, and persistence.* Unpublished master's thesis, Tufts University.

O'Connell, M., Boat, T., & Warner, K. (Eds.). (2009). *Preventing mental, emotional and behavioral disorders among young people: Progress and possibilities.* Washington, DC: National Academies Press.

Ogden, P., Minton, K., & Pain, C. (2006). *Trauma and the body: A sensorimotor approach to psychotherapy.* New York: Norton.

Pajares, F., & Schunk, D. H. (2001). Self-beliefs and school success: Self-efficacy, self concept, and school achievement. In R. Riding & S. Rayner (Eds.), *Self-perception* (pp. 239–266). Westport, CT: Ablex.

Palincsar, A. S., & Brown, A. L. (1984). Reciprocal teaching of comprehension-fostering and comprehension-monitoring activities. *Cognition and Instruction, 1*(2), 117–175.

Palincsar, A. S., Winn, J., David, Y., Snyder, B., & Stevens, D. (1993). Approaches to strategic reading instruction reflecting different assumptions regarding teaching and learning. In L. Meltzer (Ed.), *Strategy assessment and instruction for students with learning disabilities* (pp. 247–270). Austin, TX: PRO-ED.

Paris, S. G., Lipson, M., & Wixson, K. (1983). Becoming a strategic reader. *Contemporary Educational Psychology, 8*, 292–316.

Parish, P. (1963). *Amelia Bedelia.* New York: Harper & Row.

Patterson, G. R. (2002). The early development of coercive family process. In J. G. Reid, G. R Patterson, & J. Snyder (Eds.), *Antisocial behavior in children and adolescents: A developmental analysis and model for intervention* (pp. 123–145). Washington, DC: American Psychological Association.

Phillips, L. H., Bull, R., Adams, E., & Fraser, L. (2002). Positive mood and executive function: Evidence from stroop and fluency tasks. *Emotion, 2*(1), 12–22.

Pintrich, P., & Schunk, D. (1996). *Motivation in education: Theory, research and applications.* Englewood Cliffs, NJ: Prentice-Hall.

Pressley, M. (2006). *Reading instruction that works: The case for balanced teaching* (3rd ed.). New York: Guilford Press.

Pressley, M., & Afflerbach, P. (1995). *Verbal protocols of reading: The nature of constructively responsive reading.* Hillsdale, NJ: Erlbaum.

Pressley, M., Goodchild, F., Fleet, J., Zajchowski, R., & Evans, E. D. (1989). The challenges of classroom strategy instruction. *Elementary School Journal, 89,* 301–342.

Pressley, M., & Woloshyn, V. (1995). *Cognitive strategy instruction that really improves children's academic performance* (2nd ed.). Cambridge, MA: Brookline.

Ransdell, S., & Levy, C. M. (1996). Working memory constraints on writing quality and fluency. In C. M. Levy & S. Ransdell (Eds.), *The science of writing* (pp. 93–105). Mahwah, NJ: Erlbaum.

Raskind, M. H., Goldberg, R. J., Higgins, E. L., & Herman, K. L. (1999). Patterns of change and predictors of success in individuals with learning disabilities: Results from a twenty-year longitudinal study. *Learning Disability Quarterly, 19,* 70–85.

Reid, R. (1996). Research in self-monitoring with students with learning disabilities: The present, the prospects, the pitfalls. *Journal of Learning Disabilities, 29,* 317–331.

Reid, R., & Harris, K. R. (1993). Self-monitoring of attention vs. self-monitoring of performance: Effects on attention and academic performance. *Exceptional Children, 60,* 29–40.

Reid, R., & Lienemann, T. O. (2006). *Strategy instruction for students with learning disabilities.* New York: Guilford Press.

ResearchILD & Fable Vision. (2005). *Essay Express: Strategies for successful essay writing* [Computer software]. Boston: FableVision.

ResearchILD & FableVision. (2003). *BrainCogs: The personal interactive coach for learning and studying* [Computer software]. Boston: FableVision.

Reynolds, D., & Teddlie, C. (1999). *The international handbook of school effectiveness research.* London: Routledge.

Robin, A., Schneider, M., & Dolnick, M. (1976). The turtle technique: An extended case study of self-control in the classroom. *Psychology in the Schools, 13,* 449–453.

Roditi, B. N. (1993). Mathematics assessment and strategy instruction: An applied developmental approach. In L. Meltzer (Ed.), *Strategy assessment and instruction for students with learning disabilities: From theory to practice* (pp. 293–324). Austin, TX: PRO-ED.

Roditi, B. N., & Steinberg, J. (2007). The strategic math classroom: Executive function processes and mathematics learning. In L. Meltzer (Ed.), *Executive function in education: From theory to practice* (pp. 237–261). New York: Guilford Press.

Rourke, B. (Ed.). (1995). *Syndrome of nonverbal learning disabilities.* New York: Guilford Press.

Ruf, H. T., Goldsmith, H. H., Lemery-Chalfant, K., & Schmidt, N. L. (2008). Components of childhood impulsivity. *European Journal of Developmental Science, 2,* 52–76.

Ryan, R. M., & Deci, E. L. (2000). Self-determination theory and the facilitation of intrinsic motivation, social development, and well-being. *American Psychologist, 55,* 68–78.

Scanlon, D. (2002). PROVE-ing what you know: Using a learning strategy in an inclusive class. *Teaching Exceptional Children, 34*(4), 50–54.

Scardamalia, M., & Bereiter, C. (1985). Helping students become better writers. *School Administrator, 42*(4), 16–26.

Schneider, M. (1974). Turtle technique in the classroom. *Teaching Exceptional Children, 7*, 21–24.

Schroeder, M. A., & Washington, M. (1989). *Math in bloom: Multiplication/division*. East Moline, IL: LinguiSystems.

Schunk, D. H. (1980, September). *Proximal-goal facilitation of children's achievement and interest*. Paper presented at the 88th Annual Convention of the American Psychological Association, Montréal.

Schunk, D. H. (1995). Self-efficacy and education and instruction. In J. E. Maddux (Ed.), *Self efficacy, adaptation, and adjustment: Theory, research, and application* (pp. 281–303). New York: Plenum Press.

Schunk, D. H., & Swartz, C. W. (1993). Goals and progress feedback: Effects on self-efficacy and writing achievement. *Contemporary Educational Psychology, 18*(3), 337–354.

Scruggs, T. E., & Mastropieri, M. A. (2000). The effectiveness of mnemonic instruction for students with learning and behavior problems: An update and research synthesis. *Journal of Behavioral Education, 10*, 163–173.

Shanahan, C. H., & Shanahan, T. (2008). Content-area reading/learning: Flexibility in knowledge acquisition. In K. B. Cartwright (Ed.), *Literacy processes: Cognitive flexibility in learning and teaching* (pp. 208–234). New York: Guilford Press.

Shapiro, F. (1995). *Eye movement desensitization and reprocessing: Basic principles, protocols, and procedures*. New York: Guilford Press.

Shaywitz, S. (2003). *Overcoming dyslexia*. New York: Knopf.

Sheldon, K. M., & Elliot, A. J. (1999). Goal striving, need satisfaction, and longitudinal well being: The self-concordance model. *Journal of Personality and Social Psychology, 76*, 482–497.

Shimabukuro, S. M., Prater, M. A., Jenkins, A., & Edelen-Smith, P. (1999). The effects of self monitoring of academic performance on students with learning disabilities and ADD/ADHD. *Education and Treatment of Children, 22*(4), 397–415.

Siegle, P., Lange, L., & Macklem, G. (1997). *Open circle curriculum: Reach Out to Schools social competency program*. Unpublished manuscript, The Stone Center, Wellesley College.

Snow, C. E., Griffin, P., & Burns, M. S. (Eds.). (2005). *Knowledge to support the teaching of reading: Preparing teachers for a changing world*. San Francisco: Jossey-Bass.

Spector, C. C. (1997). *Saying one thing, meaning another: Activities for clarifying ambiguous language*. Eau Claire, WI: Thinking.

Spiro, R. J. (2004). Principled pluralism for adaptive flexibility in teaching and learning to read. In R. B. Ruddell & N. J. Unrau (Eds.), *Theoretical models and processes of reading* (5th ed., pp. 654–659). Newark, DE: International Reading Association.

Spiro, R. J., Feltovich, P. J., Jacobson, M. J., & Coulson, R. L. (1992). Cognitive flexibility, constructivism, and hypertext: Random access instruction for advanced knowledge acquisition in ill-structured domains. In T. M. Duffy & D. H. Jonassen (Eds.), *Constructivism and the technology of instruction* (pp. 57–75). Hillsdale, NJ: Erlbaum.

Sprenger, M. (1999). *Learning & memory: The brain in action*. Alexandria, VA: The Association for Supervision and Curriculum Development.

Stegge, H., & Terwogt, M. M. (2007). Awareness and regulation of emotion in typical and atypical development. In J. J. Gross (Ed.), *Handbook of emotion regulation* (pp. 269–286). New York: Guilford Press.

Stein, J. A., & Krishnan, K. (2007). Nonverbal learning disabilities and executive function: The challenge of effective assessment and teaching. In L. Meltzer (Ed.), *Executive function in education: From theory to practice* (pp. 106 -132). New York: Guilford Press.

Stein, J. A., Meltzer, L., Krishnan, K., Sales Pollica, L., Papadopoulos, I., & Roditi, B. (2007). *Parent guide to hassle-free homework.* New York: Scholastic.

Sternberg, R. J. (2005). Intelligence, competence, and expertise. In A. J. Elliot & C. S. Dweck (Eds.), *Handbook of competence and motivation* (pp. 15–31). New York: Guilford Press.

Stipek, D. J. (1998). *Motivation to learn: From theory to practice* (3rd ed.). Boston: Allyn & Bacon.

Stone, A. C., & Conca, L. (1993). The origin of strategy deficits in children with learning disabilities: A social constructivist perspective. In L. Meltzer (Ed.), *Strategy assessment and instruction for students with learning disabilities: From theory to practice* (pp. 23–59). Austin, TX: PRO-ED.

Stone, C. A., & May, A. (2002). The accuracy of academic self-evaluations in adolescents with learning disabilities. *Journal of Learning Disabilities, 35*(4), 370–383.

Swanson, H. L. (1989). Strategy instruction: Overview of principles and procedures for effective use. *Learning Disabilities Quarterly, 12,* 3–14.

Swanson, H. L. (1999). Instructional components that predict treatment outcomes for students with learning disabilities: Support for a combined strategy and direct instruction model. *Learning Disabilities Research and Practice, 14,* 129–140.

Swanson, H. L. (2000). Are working memory deficits in readers with learning disabilities hard to change? *Journal of Learning Disabilities, 33,* 551–566.

Swanson, H. L., Harris, K., & Graham, S. (Eds.). (2003). *Handbook of learning disabilities.* New York: Guilford Press.

Swanson, H. L., & Hoskyn, M. (1998). Experimental intervention research on students with learning disabilities: A meta-analysis of treatment outcomes. *Review of Educational Research, 68,* 277–321.

Swanson, H. L., & Hoskyn, M. (2001). Instructing adolescents with learning disabilities: A component and composite analysis. *Learning Disabilities Research and Practice, 16*(2), 109–119.

Swanson, H. L., Hoskyn, M., & Lee, C. (1999). *Interventions for students with learning disabilities: A meta-analysis of treatment outcomes.* New York: Guilford Press.

Swanson, H. L., & Sachse-Lee, C. (2001). Mathematical problem solving and working memory in children with learning disabilities: Both executive and phonological processes are important. *Journal of Experimental Child Psychology, 79*(3), 294–321.

Swanson, H. L., & Sáez, L. (2003). Memory difficulties in children and adults with learning disabilities. In H. L. Swanson, K. R. Harris, & S. Graham (Eds.), *Handbook of learning disabilities* (pp. 182–198). New York: Guilford Press.

Sweller, J., van Merrienboer, J. J., & Paas, F. G. (1998). Cognitive architecture and instructional design. *Educational Psychology Review, 10*(3), 251–296.

Tangney, J. P., Baumeister, R. F., & Boone, A. L. (2004). High self-control predicts good adjustment, less pathology, better grades, and interpersonal success. *Journal of Personality, 72,* 271–324.

Tannock, R. (Chair). (2008, March). *Inattention and working memory: Effects on academic performance.* Symposium conducted at the 23rd Annual Learning Differences Conference, Harvard Graduate School of Education, Cambridge, MA.

Taylor, C., Liang, B., Tracy, A. J., Williams, L. M., & Seigle, P. (2002). Gender differences in middle school adjustment, physical fighting and social skills: Evaluation of a social competency program. *Journal of Primary Prevention, 23*, 259–272.

Thatcher, R. W. (1997). Human frontal lobe development: A theory of cyclical cortical reorganization. In N. A. Krasnegor, G. R. Lyon, & P. S. Goldman-Rakic (Eds.), *Development of the prefrontal cortex: Evolution, neurobiology and behavior* (pp. 85–113). Baltimore: Brookes.

Thomas, A., & Chess, S. (1977). *Temperament and development.* New York: Brunner/Mazel.

Timko, M. (1998). *Reach Out to Schools: Social competency program summary of teacher training evaluations.* Unpublished manuscript, The Stone Center, Wellesley College.

Tomlinson, C. A. (1999). *The differentiated classroom: Responding to the needs of all learners.* Alexandria, VA: Association for Supervision and Curriculum Development.

Tomlinson, C. A., Brimijoin, K., & Narvaez, L. (2008). *The differentiated school: Making revolutionary changes in teaching and learning.* Alexandria, VA: Association for Supervision and Curriculum Development.

Torgesen, J. K. (1977). The role of nonspecific factors in the task performance of learning disabled children: A theoretical assessment. *Journal of Learning Disabilities, 10*, 27–34.

Torgesen, J. K. (1996). A model of memory from an information processing perspective: The special case of phonological memory. In C. R. Lyon & N. A. Krasnegor (Ed.), *Attention, memory, and executive function* (pp. 157–184). Baltimore: Brookes.

Tsai, J. L., Levenson, R. W., & McCoy, K. (2006). Cultural and temperamental variation in emotional response. *Emotion, 6*(3), 484–497.

Vail, P. (1994). *Emotions: The on/off switch for learning,* Rosemont, NJ: Modern Learning Press.

Valentine, T. (2007). Teaching transitions. *Responsive Classroom Newsletter, 19*(4), 12.

Vansteenkiste, M., Simons, J., Lens, W., Sheldon, K. M., & Deci, E. L. (2004). Motivating learning, performance, and persistence: The synergistic effects of intrinsic goal contents and autonomy-supportive contexts. *Journal of Personality and Social Psychology, 87*, 246–260.

Vener, D. (2002). *Study skills: A Landmark School student guide.* Prides Crossing, MA: Landmark School.

Vroom, V. H. (1964). *Work and motivation.* New York: Wiley.

Wagner, A. (2004). *Up and down the worry hill* (2nd ed.). Rochester, NY: Lighthouse Press.

Wagner, A. P. (2005). *Worried no more: Teaching tools and forms on CD.* Rochester, NY: Lighthouse Press.

Wagner, R. K., & Sternberg, R. J. (1987). Executive control in reading comprehension. In B. K. Britton & S. M. Glynn (Eds.), *Executive control processes in reading* (pp. 1–21). Hillsdale, NJ: Erlbaum.

Webber, J., Scheuermann, B., McCall, C., & Coleman, M. (1993). Research on self-monitoring as a behavior management technique in special education classrooms: A descriptive review. *Remedial and Special Education, 14*, 38–56.

Welch, M. (1992). The PLEASE strategy: A metacognitive learning strategy for improving the paragraph writing of students with mild disabilities. *Learning Disability Quarterly, 15*, 119–128.

Westman, A. S., & Kamoo, R. L. (1990). Relationship between using conceptual comprehension of academic material and thinking abstractly about global life issues. *Psychological Reports, 66*(2), 387–390.

White, R. W. (1959). Motivation reconsidered: The concept of competence. *Psychological Review, 66*, 297–333.

Wigfield, A., & Eccles, J. S. (2000). Expectancy-value theory of achievement motivation. *Contemporary Educational Psychology, 25*, 68–81.

Wolfe, M. B. W., & Goldman, S. R. (2005). Relationships between adolescents' text processing and reasoning. *Cognition and Instruction, 23*, 467–502.

Wolters, C. (2003). Understanding procrastination from a self-regulated learning perspective. *Journal of Educational Psychology, 95*, 179–187.

Yuill, N. (2007). Visiting Joke City: How can talking about jokes foster metalinguistic awareness in poor comprehenders? In D. MacNamara (Ed.), *Reading comprehension strategies: Theories, interventions and technologies* (pp. 325–345). New York: Erlbaum.

Yuill, N., & Bradwell, J. (1998). The laughing PC: How a software riddle package can help children's reading comprehension. *Proceedings of the British Psychological Society, 6*, 119–121.

Yuill, N., Kerawalla, L., Pearce, D., Luckin, R., & Harris, A. (2008). Using technology to teach flexibility through peer discussion. In K. B. Cartwright (Ed.), *Literacy processes: Cognitive flexibility in learning and teaching* (pp. 320–342). New York: Guilford Press.

Yun Dai, D., & Sternberg, R. J. (Eds.). (2004). *Motivation, emotion, and cognition: Integrative perspectives on intellectual functioning and development.* Mahwah, NJ: Lawrence Erlbaum.

Zelazo, P. D., & Müller, U. (2002). Executive function in typical and atypical development. In U. Goswami (Ed.), *Blackwell handbook of childhood cognitive development* (pp. 445–469). Malden, MA: Blackwell.

Zelazo, P. D., Müller, U., Frye, D., & Marcovitch, S. (2003). The development of executive function in early childhood. *Monographs of the Society for Research in Child Development, 68*(3, Serial No. 274).

Zimmerman, B. J. (1998). Academic studying and the development of personal skill: A self regulatory perspective. *Educational Psychologist, 33*, 73–86.

Zimmerman, B. J. (2000). Attaining self-regulation: A social cognitive perspective. In M. Boekaerts, P. R. Pintrich, & M. Zeidner (Eds.), *Handbook of self-regulation* (pp. 13–39). San Diego, CA: Academic Press.

Zimmerman, B. J., & Kitsantas, A. (1997). Developmental phases in self-regulation: Shifting from process to outcome goals. *Journal of Educational Psychology, 89*, 29–36.

Zimmerman, B. J., & Risemberg, R. (1997). Becoming a self-regulated writer: A social cognitive perspective. *Contemporary Educational Psychology, 22*, 73–101.

Zimmerman, B. J., & Schunk, D. H. (Eds.). (2001). *Self-regulated learning and academic achievement: Theoretical perspectives* (2nd ed.). Mahwah, NJ: Erlbaum.

Zins, J. E., Bloodworth, M. R., Weissberg, R. P., & Walberg, H. J. (2004). The scientific base linking social and emotional learning to school success. In J. E. Zins, R. P. Weissberg, M. C. Wang, & H. J. Walberg (Eds.), *Building academic success on social and emotional learning: What does the research say?* New York: Teachers College Press.

Zins, J. E., Weissberg, R. P., Wang, M. C., & Walberg, H. J. (Eds.) (2004). *Building academic success on social and emotional learning: What does the research say?* New York: Teachers College Press.

Index

Page numbers followed by an *f* or a *t* indicate figures or tables.